T0389463

Shoulder Instability

Giovanni Di Giacomo • Alberto Costantini • Andrea De Vita • Nicola de Gasperis
Editors

Shoulder Instability

Alternative Surgical Techniques

Forewords by
James C. Esch
Gilles Walch

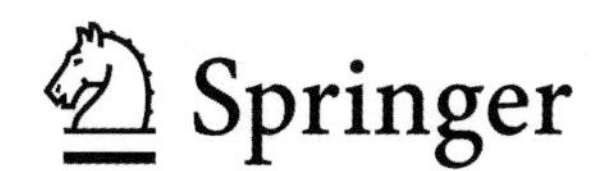

Giovanni Di Giacomo
Arthroscopic Surgery Department
Concordia Hospital for Special Surgery
Rome, Italy

Alberto Costantini
Arthroscopic Surgery Department
Concordia Hospital for Special Surgery
Rome, Italy

Andrea De Vita
Arthroscopic Surgery Department
Concordia Hospital for Special Surgery
Rome, Italy

Nicola de Gasperis
Arthroscopic Surgery Department
Concordia Hospital for Special Surgery
Rome, Italy

Library of Congress Control Number: 2011926813

ISBN 978-88-470-2034-4 e-ISBN 978-88-470-2035-1

DOI 10.1007/978-88-470-2035-1

Springer Milan Dordrecht Heidelberg London New York

Cover design: Ikona S.r.l., Milan, Italy
Typesetting: C & G di Cerri e Galassi, Cremona, Italy
Printing and binding: Grafiche Porpora, Segrate (MI), Italy

Printed in Italy

Springer-Verlag Italia S.r.l., Via Decembrio 28, I-20137 Milano
Springer is part of Springer Science+Business Media (www.springer.com)

I dedicate this book to all my patients for their trust in me and the opportunities they have offered me over many years.

Giovanni Di Giacomo

To my mentors Giovanni, Alberto, and Andrea. To my parents, and to my wife, Virginia.

Nicola de Gasperis

To my mother Florinda, my father Gelsomino, and my brother Francesco.

Andrea De Vita

I would like to thank my family: Giusy, Andrea, Stefano, and my mother and father for their help and understanding.

Alberto Costantini

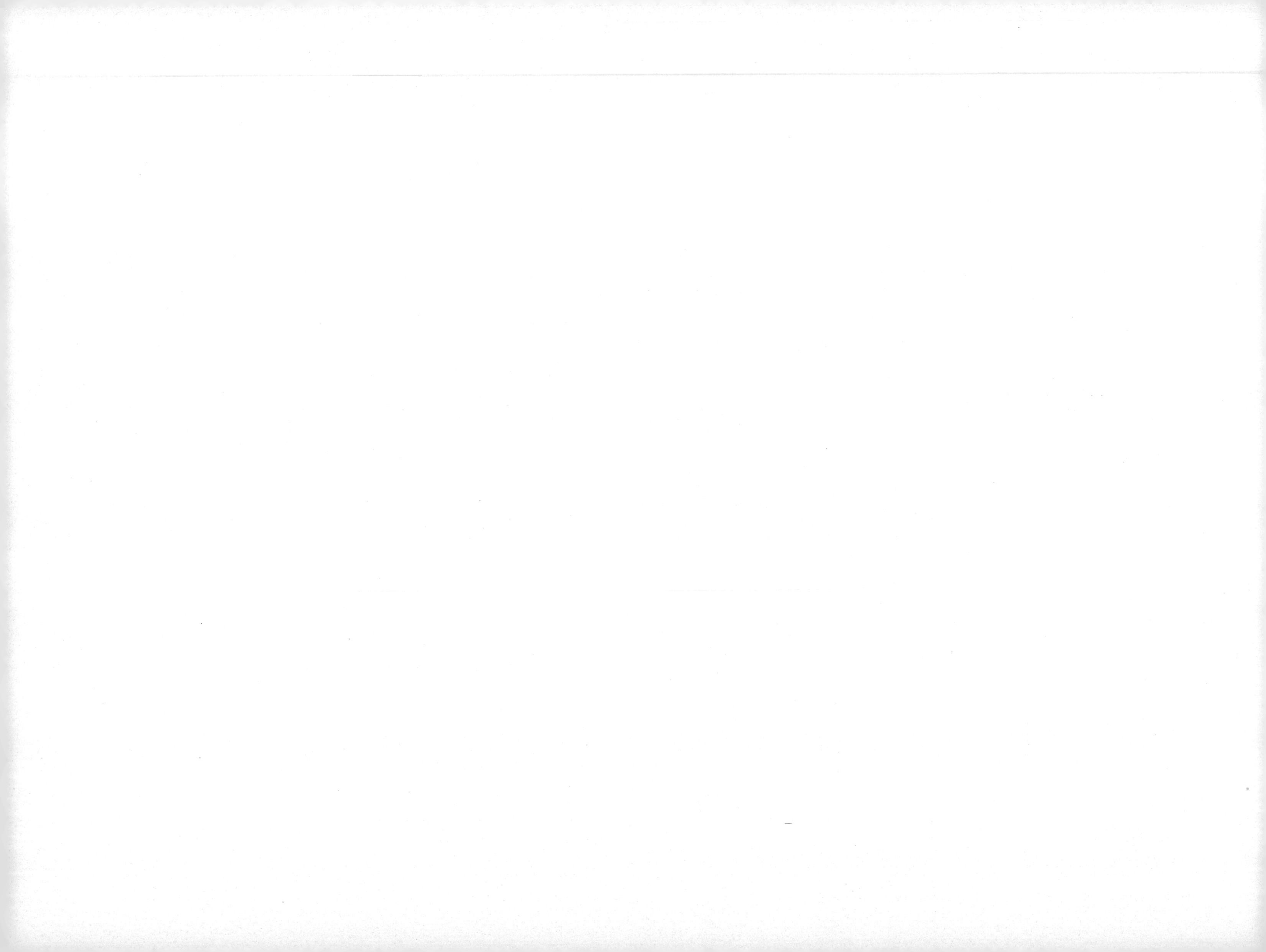

Foreword

Arthroscopic instability surgery has created a generation of surgeons who can repair an unstable shoulder by fixing a labrum to bone with suture anchors. Unfortunately, the failure rate ranges from 10% to 40%, especially in young active individuals. Engaging bone loss on both the humeral and glenoid sides as the arm is moved through a range of motion is often the reason for failure. This book offers surgical solutions to this often unappreciated bone loss. Giovanni Di Giacomo treats the reader to a beautifully illustrated, modern update of traditional procedures that address this difficult problem.

Each chapter is authored by experienced surgeons and provides a detailed understanding of the glenoid track as the large humeral ball with a defect moves on the smaller glenoid with bone loss. This is similar to a dented ping-pong ball moving on a golf tee that has a broken edge. Secure glenoid-rim bone-loss repair and fixation is detailed with a choice of using either the coracoid, iliac crest, or distal tibia allograft. Indications and options for humeral fixation range from filling the Hill-Sachs defect with bone to a resurfacing prosthesis. The renewed description of the traditional open surgical repair using, instead, a double-row capsular technique, is particularly interesting.

Shoulder Instability: Alternative Surgical Techniques is a welcome addition to the shoulder surgeon's armamentarium, contributing to awareness for recognizing and treating this difficult problem. Our patients will welcome better results.

James C. Esch, M.D.
Orthopaedic Specialists of North County
Oceanside, CA, USA

Foreword

The Italian School of Orthopedic Surgery has a long history related to addressing anterior shoulder instability (Putti, Delitala). For 20 years, Giovanni Di Giacomo has been an Italian pioneer of the new era of arthroscopic shoulder stabilization. His work is particularly dedicated to the difficult problem of treating athletes.

Arthroscopic treatment failure is observed in cases of severe bony defects, and it is often after such failure that the surgeon is faced with a difficult dilemma: should the glenoid-bone defect, the humeral defect, or both be treated? Giovanni Di Giacomo, Alberto Costantini, Andrea De Vita, and Nicola de Gasperis present an outstanding collection of surgical techniques by renowned surgeons addressing severe bony defects of the humerus and glenoid.

Di Giacomo and colleagues describe their precise technique of open Latarjet procedure, placing the coracoid with the patient in the lying position and fixing it with two screws and a new ingenious plate to distribute constraints and avoid coracoid nonunion or fracture. Matthew Provencher and colleagues propose two different techniques: the first is an intra-articular bone graft with the tricortical iliac crest contoured to re-establish glenoid cavity and width; the second, original and previously unpublished, uses an allograft of the distal lateral aspect of the tibia that, interestingly, matches the curvature and concavity of the native glenoid. Dario Petriccioli and colleagues propose a modified Eden-Hybbinette procedure using an autogenous tricortical iliac-crest bone graft to compensate for defects involving approximately 30% or more of the glenoid articular surface. Herbert Resch and colleagues propose their J-bone-graft technique to treat bony defects exceeding the width of the rim cortex. A wedge-shaped bone block is harvested from the iliac crest, carefully modelled, and fitted into a preformed crevice of the glenoid neck. Fixation is achieved by impaction, and no metallic screw is used. David Altchek and coworkers describe a beautiful technique with soft tissue repair only. This double-row capsulolabral repair eliminates the need to compensate for the bone defect.

Humeral defects have been analyzed since reports by Malgaigne in the 1830s and Hill and Sachs in the 1940s. Eiji Itoi and colleagues developed an intriguing approach to this defect and describe their new concept of the glenoid track with the purpose of evaluating the size of the Hill-Sachs lesion and glenoid. The glenoid track is a contact zone of the glenoid on the humeral head with the arm at the end range of motion. This approach makes it easier to understand when and how the engaging Hill-Sachs lesion can be considered a main cause of recurrent instability. Anthony Miniaci and Pradeep Kodali propose an original technique to address Hill-Sachs lesions by focal resurfacing of a humeral-head defect with a HemiCAP arthroplasty.

Each technique is meticulously described with the same spirit and plan of helping the orthopedic surgeon to perform it accurately and safely. For each step, the authors provide tips and tricks to facilitate the procedure, as well as possible complications and solutions to address them. Each chapter is richly illustrated with intraoperative color images of each step.

Di Giacomo brought together a talented group of shoulder specialists and must be commended for the exceptional quality of this textbook and congratulated for a job well done. This book will be valuable to all shoulder surgeons facing patients with recurrent anterior shoulder instability with bony defect.

Docteur Gilles Walch
Chirurgien orthopédiste
Département de Chirurgie de l'épaule
Centre Orthopédique Santy
Hopital Privé Jean Mermoz
Lyon, France

Preface

Shoulder arthroscopy is an instrument of undisputable success, but the intense use of the technique in recent years, in particular to correct shoulder instability, has revealed limitations that have become the focus of ongoing discussion.

Attention must be given to selecting the surgical patient and correctly interpreting anatomical lesions (bone loss, glenoid track, tissue quality), which seems to be taking us back to open techniques that, perhaps, we began to consider "old" too early.

With the aid of a pool of international experts, this book reviews some of these techniques, which represent a valid alternative to surgical arthroscopy and its failures. We trust it will encourage both younger and older surgeons to return, where necessary, to those procedures that must not be forgotten but, on the contrary, are crucial for the cultural and technical background of those who deal with shoulder pathologies.

Giovanni Di Giacomo

Contents

Chapter 3 - Latarjet Procedure: the Miniplate Surgical Technique

Giovanni Di Giacomo, Alberto Costantini, Andrea De Vita and Nicola de Gasperis

Chapter 4 - Double-Row Capsulolabral Repair

Craig S. Mauro, Sommer Hammoud, Courtney K. Dawson and David W. Altchek

Chapter 5 - The J-Bone Graft for Anatomical Reconstruction of Glenoid Defects

Alexander Auffarth, Mark Tauber and Herbert Resch

Chapter 6 - Iliac-crest Graft and Distal Tibia Allograft Procedure

Matthew T. Provencher, Andrew R. Hsu, Neil S. Ghodadra and Anthony A. Romeo

Chapter 8 - Focal Resurfacing of Humeral-head Defects

Pradeep Kodali, Anthony Miniaci

Contributors

David W. Altchek
Sports Medicine and Shoulder Service, Hospital for Special Surgery, New York, USA

Alexander Auffarth
Department of General Traumatology and Sports Injuries, Paracelsus Medical University, Salzburg, Austria

Paolo Baudi
Department of Orthopaedics, Ramazzini Hospital, Carpi (Mo), Italy

Celeste Bertone
Department of Orthopaedic Surgery, "Città di Brescia" Clinical Institute, Brescia, Italy

Alberto Costantini
Arthroscopic Surgery Department, Concordia Hospital for Special Surgery, Rome, Italy

Courtney K. Dawson
Sports Medicine and Shoulder Service, Hospital for Special Surgery, New York, USA

Nicola de Gasperis
Arthroscopic Surgery Department, Concordia Hospital for Special Surgery, Rome, Italy

Andrea De Vita
Arthroscopic Surgery Department, Concordia Hospital for Special Surgery, Rome, Italy

Giovanni Di Giacomo
Arthroscopic Surgery Department, Concordia Hospital for Special Surgery, Rome, Italy

Neil S. Ghodadra
Department of Orthopaedic Surgery, Rush University Medical Center, Chicago, IL, USA

Sommer Hammoud
Sports Medicine and Shoulder Service, Hospital for Special Surgery, New York, USA

Andrew R. Hsu
Department of Orthopaedic Surgery, Rush University Medical Center, Chicago, IL, USA

Eiji Itoi
Department of Orthopaedic Surgery, Tohoku University School of Medicine, Sendai, Japan

Pradeep Kodali
Department of Orthopaedic Surgery, University of Texas Health Science Center, Houston, TX, USA

Giacomo Marchi
Department of Orthopaedic Surgery, "Città di Brescia" Clinical Institute, Brescia, Italy

Craig S. Mauro
University of Pittsburgh Medical Center, UPMC St. Margaret, Pittsburgh, Pennsylvania, USA

Giuseppe Milano
Department of Orthopaedics, Università Cattolica, Rome, Italy

Anthony Miniaci
Orthopaedic Surgery – Sports Health, Cleveland Clinic Foundation, Ohio, USA

Yasushi Omori
Department of Orthopaedic Surgery, Tohoku University School of Medicine, Sendai, Japan

Dario Petriccioli
Department of Orthopaedic Surgery, "Città di Brescia" Clinical Institute, Brescia, Italy

Matthew T. Provencher
Shoulder, Knee and Sports Surgery, Department of Orthopaedic Surgery, Naval Medical Center San Diego,
San Diego, CA, USA

Herbert Resch
Department of General Traumatology and Sports Injuries, Paracelsus Medical University, Salzburg, Austria

Paolo Righi
Department of Orthopaedics, San Camillo Hospital, Forte Dei Marmi, Italy

Anthony A. Romeo
Department of Orthopaedic Surgery, Rush University Medical Center, Chicago, IL, USA

Eugenio Rossi Urtoler
Department of Orthopaedics, Ramazzini Hospital, Carpi (Mo), Italy

Mark Tauber
Department of General Traumatology and Sports Injuries, Paracelsus Medical University, Salzburg, Austria

Nobuyuki Yamamoto
Department of Orthopaedic Surgery, Tohoku University School of Medicine, Sendai, Japan

Chapter 1 – Glenoid Track

Eiji Itoi, Noboyuki Yamamoto and Yasushi Omori

1.1 Classification of Shoulder Instability

There are two distinct types of shoulder instability: 1) traumatic unilateral instability often with a Bankart lesion and usually requiring surgery (TUBS), and 2) atraumatic, multidirectional laxity, frequently bilateral, responds well to rehabilitation, however, should surgery be performed, an inferior capsular shift procedure is the treatment of choice (AMBRI) [1]. Whereas this classification does not include all types of instability, it does include the two most common types. Another classification that is important to understand is the one based on the position of the shoulder: midrange and end-range instability [2]. When the shoulder is in the mid-range of motion, all capsuloligamentous structures are lax and thus play no role as stabilizers. In this position, the shoulder is stabilized either by the negative intra-articular pressure (hanging-arm position without muscle contraction) or by the concavity-compression effect caused by the muscle contraction force against the glenoid concavity [3]. Any pathology that causes insufficiency in the mid-range stabilizers will cause mid-range instability. For example, if there is a large bony glenoid defect, the concavity-compression effect cannot be fully created, resulting in mid-range instability. Muscle imbalance, which makes it difficult to keep the humeral head centered in the glenoid socket, or enlarged joint volume with a thin joint capsule, which makes it difficult to keep the negative intra-articular pressure, also causes mid-range instability. On the other hand, when the shoulder is at the limit of motion, e.g., in abduction and maximum external rotation and maximum horizontal extension, the anteroinferior capsule becomes tight and plays a role as a stabilizer. This end-range stability deteriorates if there is disruption of the anteroinferior capsule, such as a Bankart lesion. A large Hill-Sachs lesion, which engages with the anterior rim of the glenoid at the end range of motion, is also related to end-range but not to mid-range instability. This concept is very important in order to properly understand the pathophysiology associated with bony defect of the glenoid and the humeral head.

1.2 Algorithm of Treatment

There are various treatment options for the first-time traumatic dislocation of the shoulder. Immobilization in internal rotation has been a standard treatment. However, the recurrence rate could not be reduced with increased rigidity or increased length of immobilization [4]. A new method of immobilization with the arm in external rotation is reported to be more effective in terms of reducing the recurrence rate [5]. There are a few randomized clinical trials reported with positive [6] and negative [7, 8] results. One explanation may be the brace. Some braces are not as efficient as others in keeping the arm in external rotation [9]. The ability of the brace to keep the arm in the intended position is critical. Nagaraj and colleagues used a cast to keep the immobilization position, which is probably the most secure means [6]. This may be the reason their results were superior. Other possible explanations are sample size or how soon the shoulders were immobilized after injury. This treatment, however, is not finalized. Immobilization position and period need to be further studied.

The more dislocation recurs, the more damage occurs in the shoulder joint. This is the reason some doctors recommend stabilization surgery after the initial dislocation [10–13]. However, the number needed to treat for surgical treatment is calculated to be 3.2 [14]. This means if all initial dislocations are treated surgically, two of three patients would undergo unnecessary surgery. In order to avoid this overtreatment, it may be wise to wait for the second dislocation to occur. According to the meta-analysis, there is no difference in recurrence or complication rates between those surgically treated after the initial dislocation and those surgically treated after the second or more dislocations [15]. On the other hand, patients, especially in-season athletes, wish to return to sports as soon as possible. For this purpose, various kinds of protective braces are available. The basic concept of these braces is to limit shoulder motion to prevent abduction and maximum external rotation (apprehension position). Recurrence rate with this protective brace is 38% [16]. Based upon these data, my treatment algorithm is as follows (Fig. 1.1). For

Fig. 1.1. Treatment algorithm. *Immob*, immobilization; *ER*, external rotation

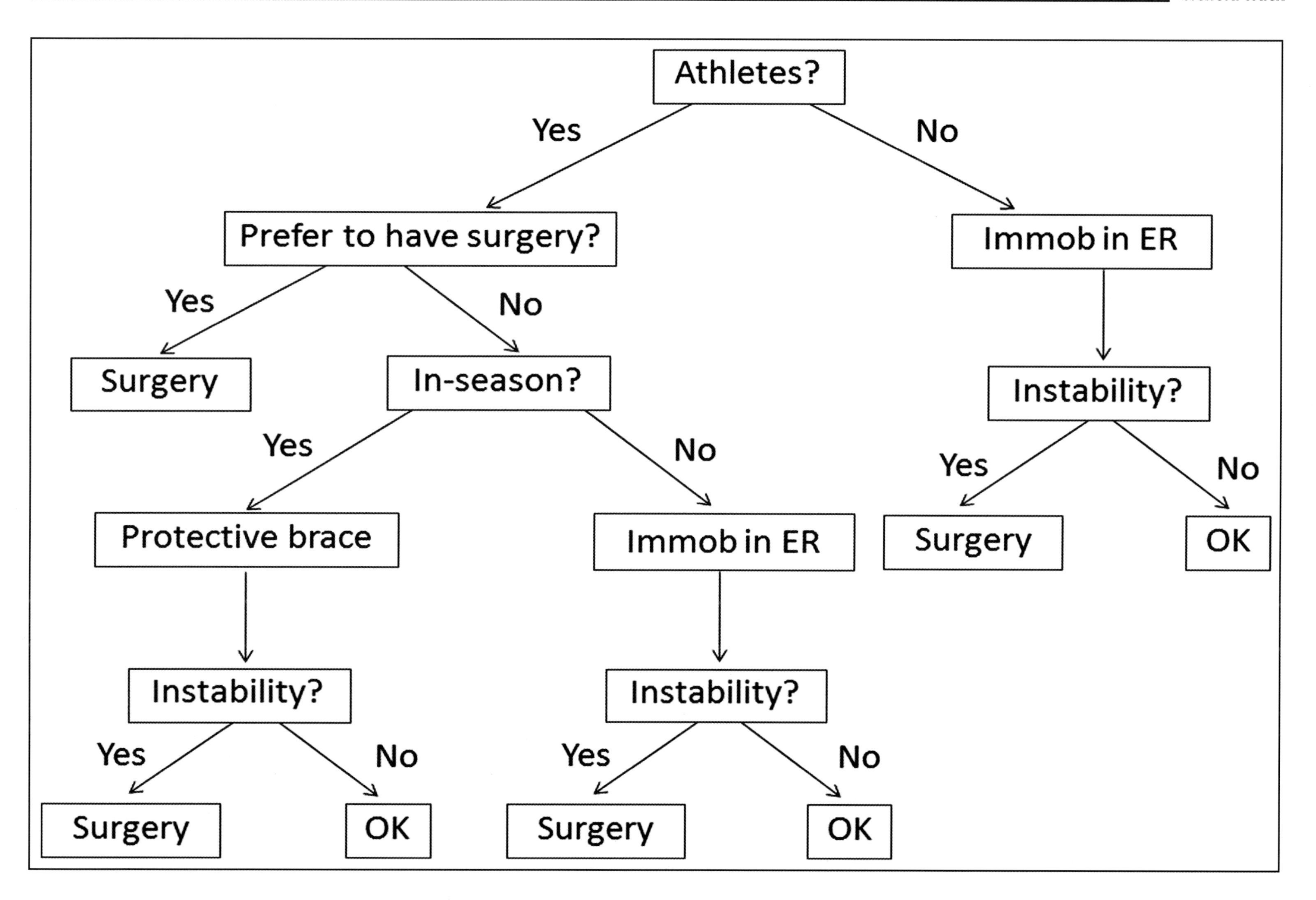
Athletes?
Yes
No
Prefer to have surgery?
Immob in ER
Yes
No
Surgery
In-season?
Instability?
Yes
No
Yes
No
Protective brace
Immob in ER
Surgery
OK
Instability?
Instability?
Yes
No
Yes
No
Surgery
OK
Surgery
OK

in-season athletes, I recommend a protective brace and consider surgical stabilization if the shoulder is unstable after the season.

1.3 Hill-Sachs Lesion

Shoulders with primary or recurrent anterior dislocations often have bony lesions of the glenoid and the humeral head. Bony lesions of the glenoid are observed in 90% of shoulders with recurrent anterior dislocations [17]. A humeral-head lesion, a compression fracture created by the anterior rim of the glenoid when the humeral head is dislocated, is observed in 47–93% of shoulders after a first-time dislocation [18–21] and 77–93% of shoulders with recurrent dislocations [19, 20, 22–24]. The Hill-Sachs lesion is located between 0 mm and 24 mm from the top of the humeral head [25]. Below this level, the Hill-Sachs lesion overlaps with the bare area of humeral head. On the clock face with the bicipital groove as 12 o'clock, the Hill-Sachs lesion is pointing toward 7:58 on average (6:46 at the top and 8:56 at the bottom).

1.4 Surgical Indication for Hill-Sachs Lesion

As mentioned previously, a Hill-Sachs lesion may cause instability with the arm at the end range of motion. If the lesion is wider than the glenoid at the end range of motion, the anterior rim of the glenoid engages with the lesion and causes another dislocation at this position. On the other hand, as the lesion shifts away from the anterior rim of the glenoid in the mid-range of motion, there is no risk of engagement and dislocation. A Hill-Sachs lesion that is covered by the glenoid socket at the end range of motion is safe because there is no risk of dislocation (Fig. 1.2). However, the same lesion is

Fig. 1.2. Relative size of the Hill-Sachs lesion. This lesion (*arrowheads*) is entirely covered by the intact glenoid (*curved arrow*) at the end range of motion. There is no risk of engagement between the glenoid and the lesion

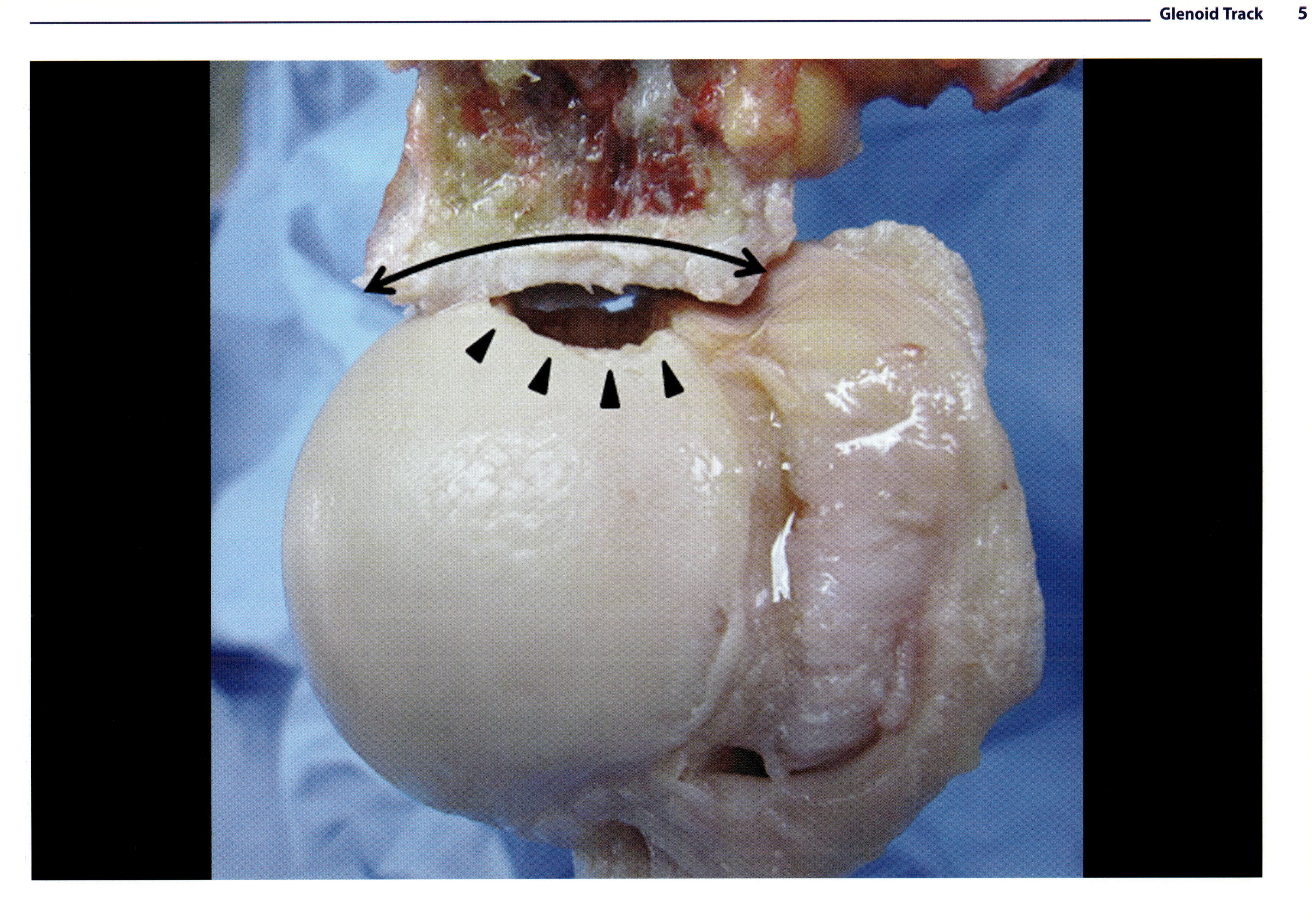

no longer safe if there is a bony defect of the glenoid and the deficient glenoid cannot cover the lesion (Fig. 1.3). In other words, whether a Hill-Sachs lesion is safe or not depends on the size of the lesion relative to the glenoid size, not on the absolute size of the lesion alone.

However, all previous reports regarding the indication of the Hill-Sachs lesion deal with lesion size alone: a Hill-Sachs lesion needs to be treated when it is large (≥4.0 cm × 1.0 cm) or medium-sized (4.0 cm × 0.5 cm) [26], when it is >20% [27] or 25% [28] of the humeral head, when its depth is >16% of the humeral head diameter, or when its volume is >1,000 mm^3 [29]. All these investigators reported the indication determined by the size of the Hill-Sachs lesion alone, and none took the size of the glenoid into consideration.

Fig. 1.3. Relative size of the Hill-Sachs lesion. The same lesion (*arrowheads*) cannot be entirely covered by the glenoid with an anterior rim defect (*white arrows*). There is a risk of engagement between the glenoid and the lesion

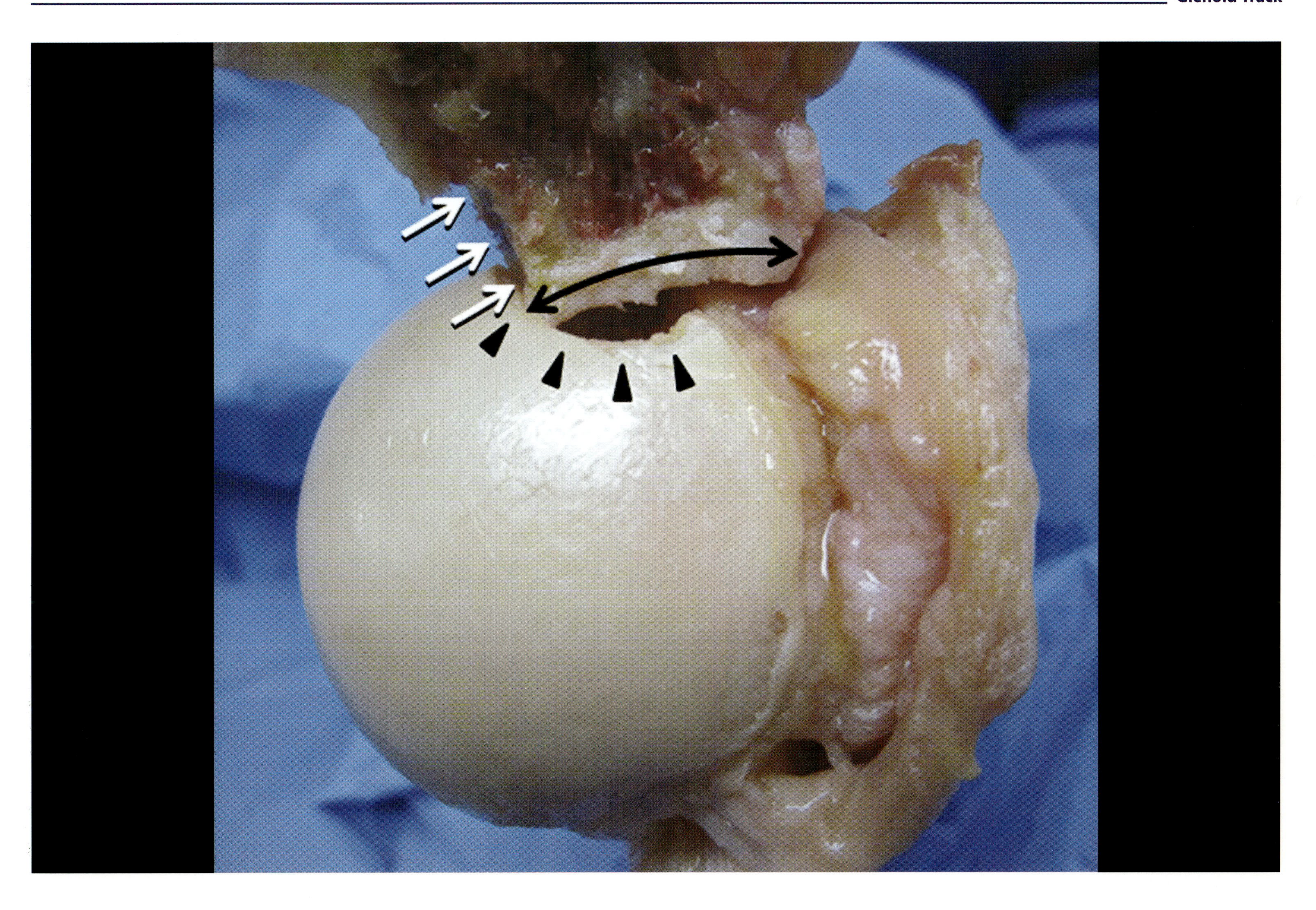

1.5. Glenoid Track

1.5.1 A New Concept

For the purpose of evaluating the size of the Hill-Sachs lesion together with the size of the glenoid, we introduced a new concept: the glenoid track [30]. The glenoid track is a contact zone of the glenoid on the humeral head with the arm at the end range of motion, e.g., in various degrees of elevation with the arm in maximum external rotation and maximum horizontal extension. This end range of motion is critical for anterior dislocation because the anterior soft tissue structures become tight and prevent the anterior translation of the humeral head in this position. It is this position that patients with recurrent anterior dislocation of the shoulder feel anterior apprehension. If the Hill-Sachs lesion is always covered by the glenoid at this end range of motion, or in other words, if the Hill-Sachs lesion stays within the glenoid track, the lesion does no harm, because it is always covered by the glenoid even at the end range of motion. On the other hand, if the lesion comes out of the glenoid coverage, it engages with the anterior rim of the glenoid and causes a dislocation. Clarifying the exact location of this contact zone or the glenoid track enables us to evaluate any Hill-Sachs lesion for its risk of engagement.

1.5.2 Glenoid Track in Cadaveric Shoulders

First, we used cadaveric shoulders to determine where the glenoid track was. The scapula was fixed on the fixator while the arm was elevated from 0° to 60° relative to the scapula (90° relative to the trunk), with the arm in maximum external rotation and horizontal extension. The position of the glenoid rim was marked on the articular cartilage of the humeral head with the arm elevated at 0°, 30°, and 60° relative to the scapula, which were equivalent to 0°, 45°, and 90° of elevation relative to the trunk. As the arm was elevated along the end range of motion, the glenoid moved from inferomedial to superolateral portion of the humeral head, along the posterior margin of the articular surface of the humeral head (Fig. 1.4). During this movement, the glenoid created a zone of contact with the humeral head (Fig. 1.5). This zone of contact is the glenoid track. As long as the Hill-Sachs lesion is within this track, there is no chance that the anterior rim of the glenoid

Fig. 1.4. Position of the glenoid. The glenoid rim was marked on the articular surface of the humeral head with the arm at 0° (*green dots*), 30° (*blue dots*), and 60° (*red dots*) of abduction

Fig. 1.5. Glenoid track. The contact area of the glenoid on the humeral head when the arm was moved along the end range of motion was defined as the glenoid track (*yellow zone*)

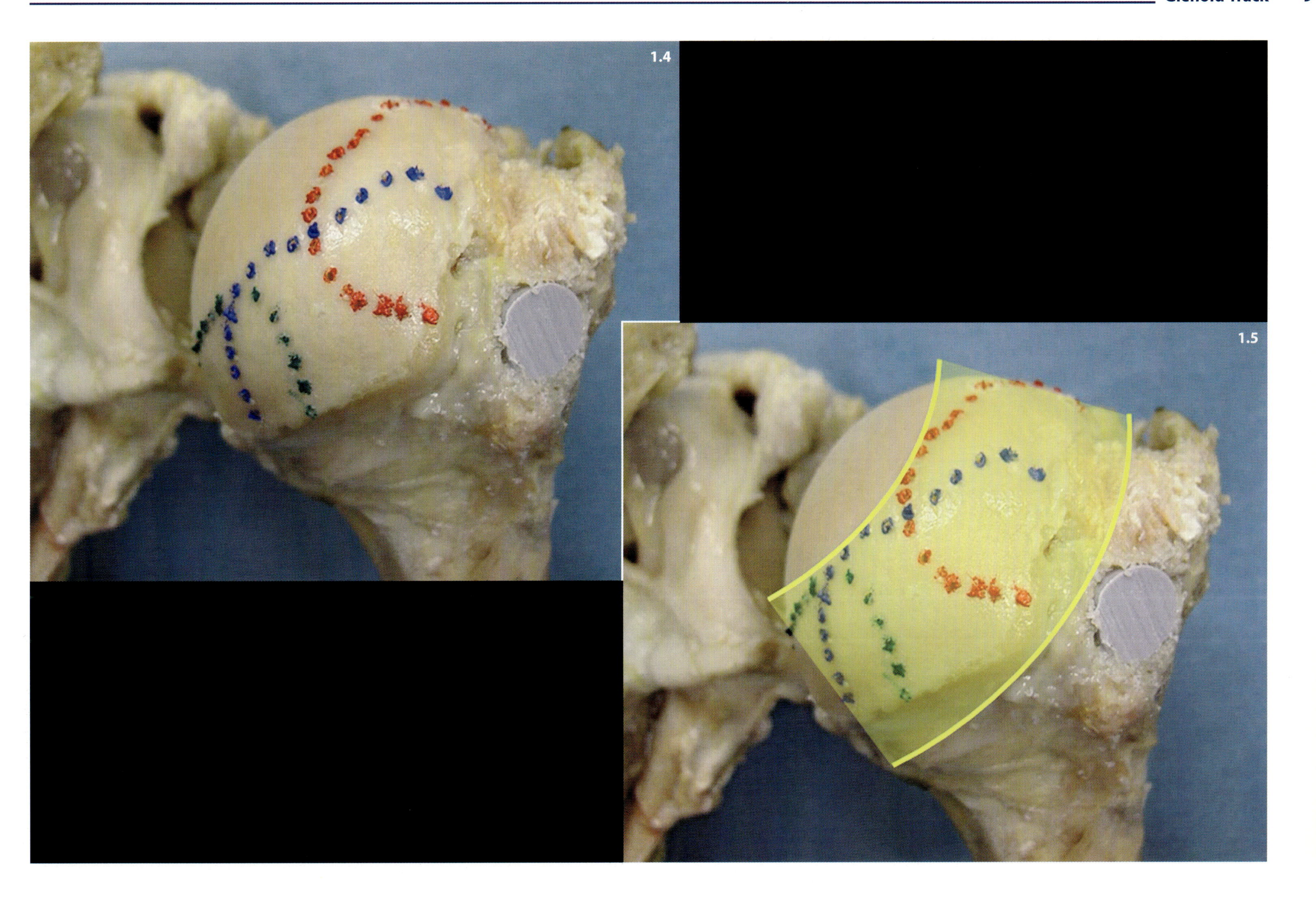
1.4
1.5

(medial margin of the glenoid track) engages with the Hill-Sachs lesion (Fig. 1.6). If the lesion extends further over the medial margin of the glenoid track, then there is a risk of engagement and dislocation at this point where the lesion crosses over the medial margin of the glenoid track (Fig. 1.7). The location of the medial margin of the glenoid track, therefore, is very crucial in terms of evaluating the risk of a Hill-Sachs lesion causing engagement and dislocation. We measured the width of the glenoid and found that with the arm at 90° of abduction, the medial margin of the glenoid track was located at the distance equivalent to 84% of the

Fig. 1.6. Hill-Sachs lesion inside the glenoid track. The medial margin of the glenoid track represents the trace of the anterior rim of the glenoid. In this case, the lesion (*dark blue semicircular area*) is located more lateral than the medial margin of the glenoid track, which means that there is no chance that this lesion engages with the anterior rim of the glenoid

Fig. 1.7. Hill-Sachs lesion out of the glenoid track. In this case, the lesion (*dark blue semicircular area*) extends more medially over the medial margin of the glenoid track. At this cross-over, there is a risk of engagement between the glenoid and the lesion

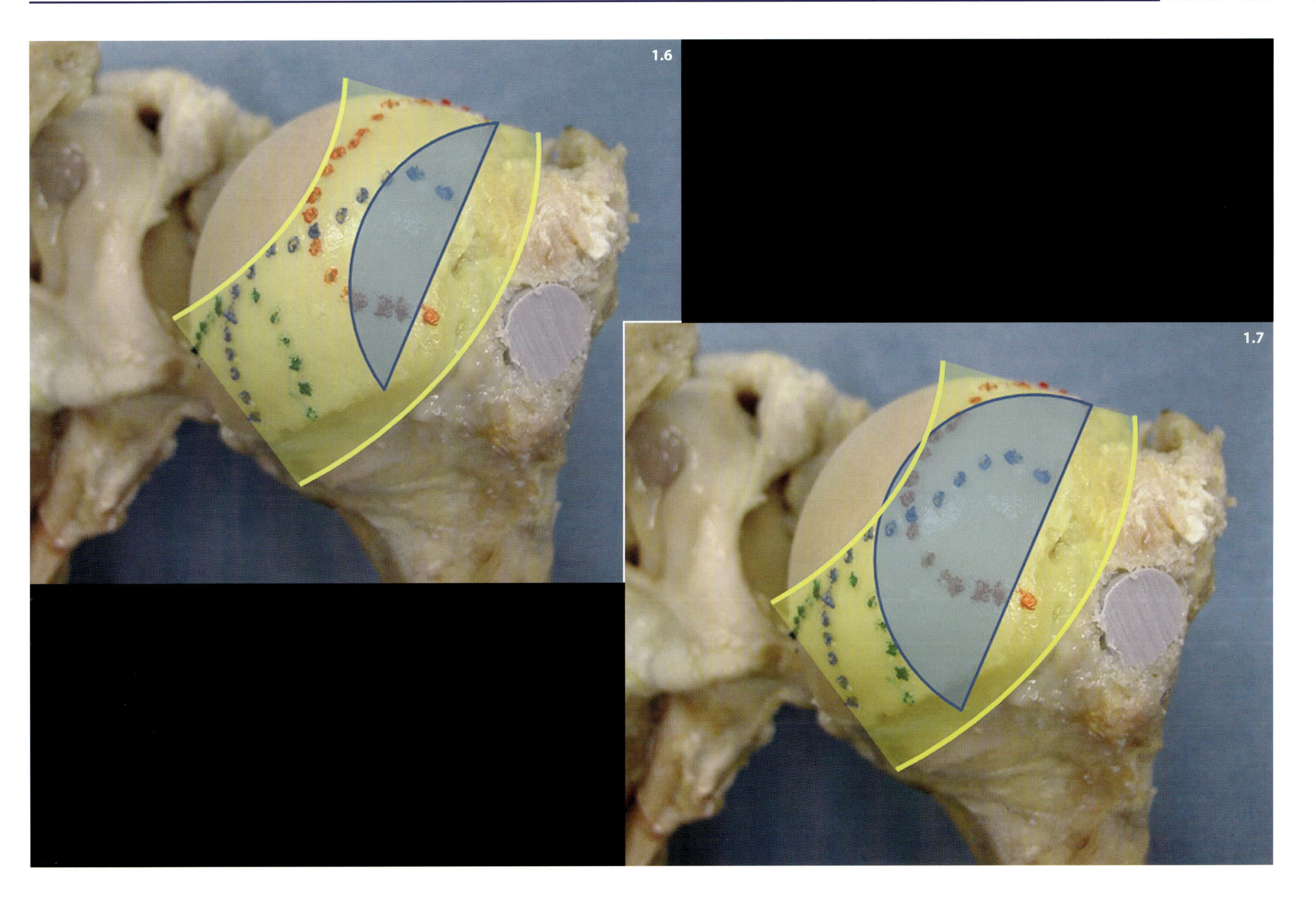
1.6
1.7

glenoid width from the medial margin of the footprint of the rotator cuff (Fig. 1.8).

1.5.3 Glenoid Track in Live Shoulders

Next, we measured the glenoid track in live shoulders using healthy volunteers [31]. Magnetic resonance imaging (MRI) was taken at seven different angles of arm elevation while the arm was kept in maximum external rotation and horizontal extension. Using the motion analysis system created by Sugamoto of Osaka University School of Medicine, Osaka, Japan, three-dimensional models of the scapula and humerus were created from MRI data. Then, scapula and humerus movements were calculated by voxel-based registration of each model. Finally, the humeral head was fixed, and glenoid movement during this end range of motion was visualized. For the purpose of measuring the position of the glenoid track, glenoid positions at 60°, 90°,

Fig. 1.8. Location of the glenoid track. The medial margin of the glenoid track is located at a distance equivalent to 84% of the glenoid width from the footprint of the rotator cuff (*dotted line*)

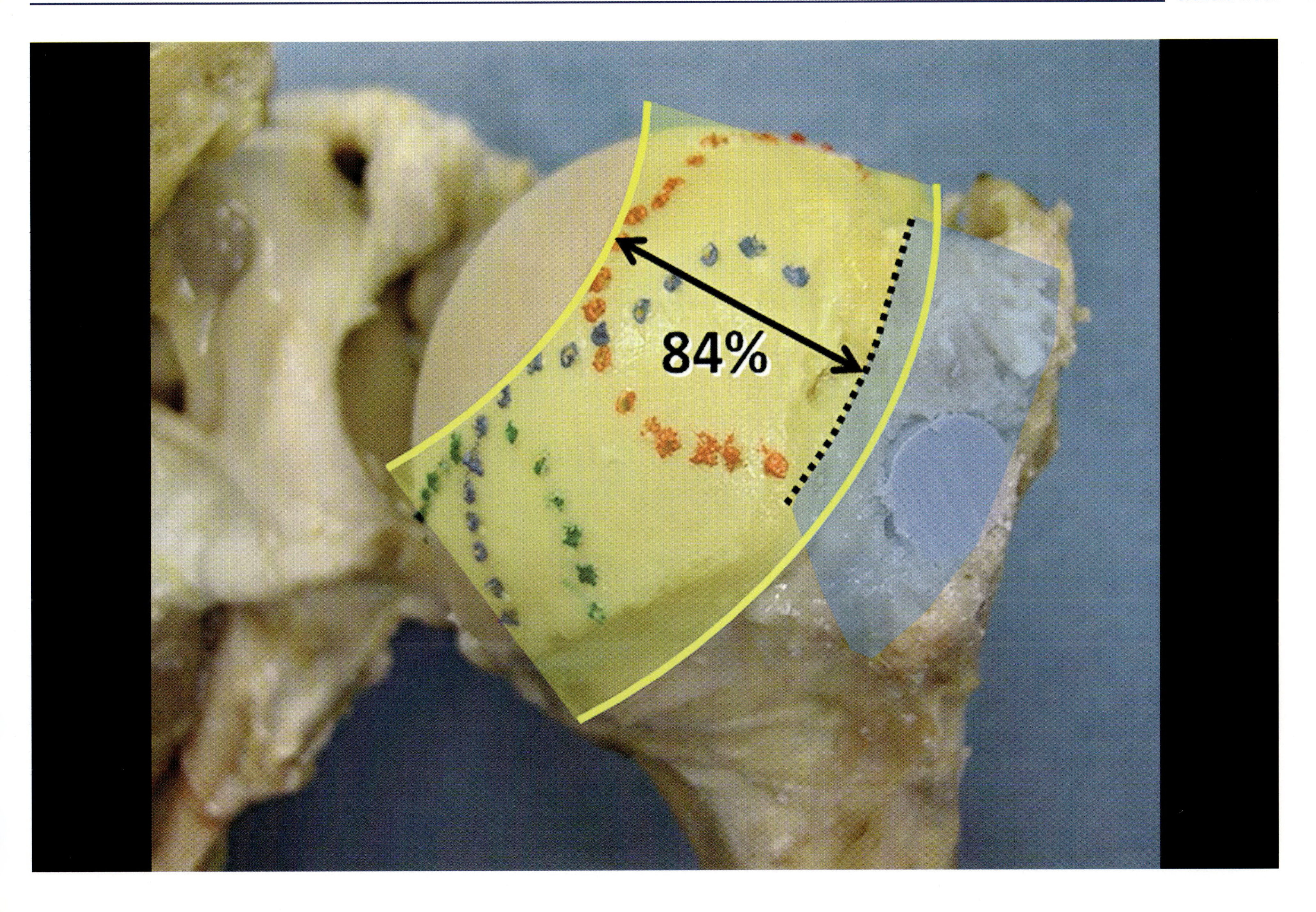
84%

120°, and 150° of elevation were overimposed on the humeral head (Fig. 1.9). The location of the medial margin of the glenoid track was calculated to be 93%, 85%, 82%, and 82% with the arm at 60°, 90°, 120°, and 150° of elevation, respectively (Fig. 1.10). This value at 90° of elevation is very close to that obtained in cadaveric shoulders.

1.5.4 Clinical Application

We can now evaluate every Hill-Sachs lesion for its risk of engagement using this glenoid track concept. As the glenoid moves on the lesion when the arm is moving along the end range of motion, any obstacle attached to the lesion would prevent the smooth movement of the glenoid. For example, the remplissage technique is becoming increasingly popular [32]. With this procedure, the infraspinatus tendon is fixed into the cavity of the lesion. Obviously, the fixed tendon prevents smooth movement of the glenoid over the lesion, thus creating a limited range of motion. This may not be problematic during activities of daily living because this limitation occurs at the end range of motion. However, for a throwing athlete, this limitation could be critical. When using this technique, it is important to carefully assess the activity levels of each patient beforehand.

1.6 Surgical Procedures for Hill-Sachs Lesion

Treatment strategy for a large Hill-Sachs lesion that extends medially over the glenoid track is either to: 1) fill the lesion defect or 2) limit the external rotation to avoid engagement. Filling the defect avoids further engagement because there is no defect to engage. This can be achieved either by bone grafting [27, 28], transhumeral head plasty [33, 34], or soft tissue transfer such as reverse McLaughlin procedure [35] or remplissage [32]. Theoretically, bone grafting does not cause any limitation in the range of motion, but remplissage does, as described above. Limiting the external rotation can be achieved by rotational humeral osteotomy [36] or by tightening the anterior soft tissue structures such as in Magnuson-Stack and Putti-Platt procedures [37]. According to Burkhart and De Beer [38], 21 of 194 (10.8%) patients had significant bony defects (three Hill-Sachs and 18 bony glenoid defects). Although not as common as they may be, these cases with significant bony defects need to be selected and treated properly to avoid remnant instability.

Fig. 1.9. Glenoid track in live shoulders. *Red dots* indicate the most medial portion of the glenoid at 60°, 90°, 120°, and 150° of abduction from bottom to top

Fig. 1.10. Glenoid track in live shoulders. Average locations of these dots from the medial margin of the footprint of the rotator cuff (*dotted line*) are 93% of the glenoid width at 60° of abduction, 85% at 90°, 82% at 120°, and 82% at 150°

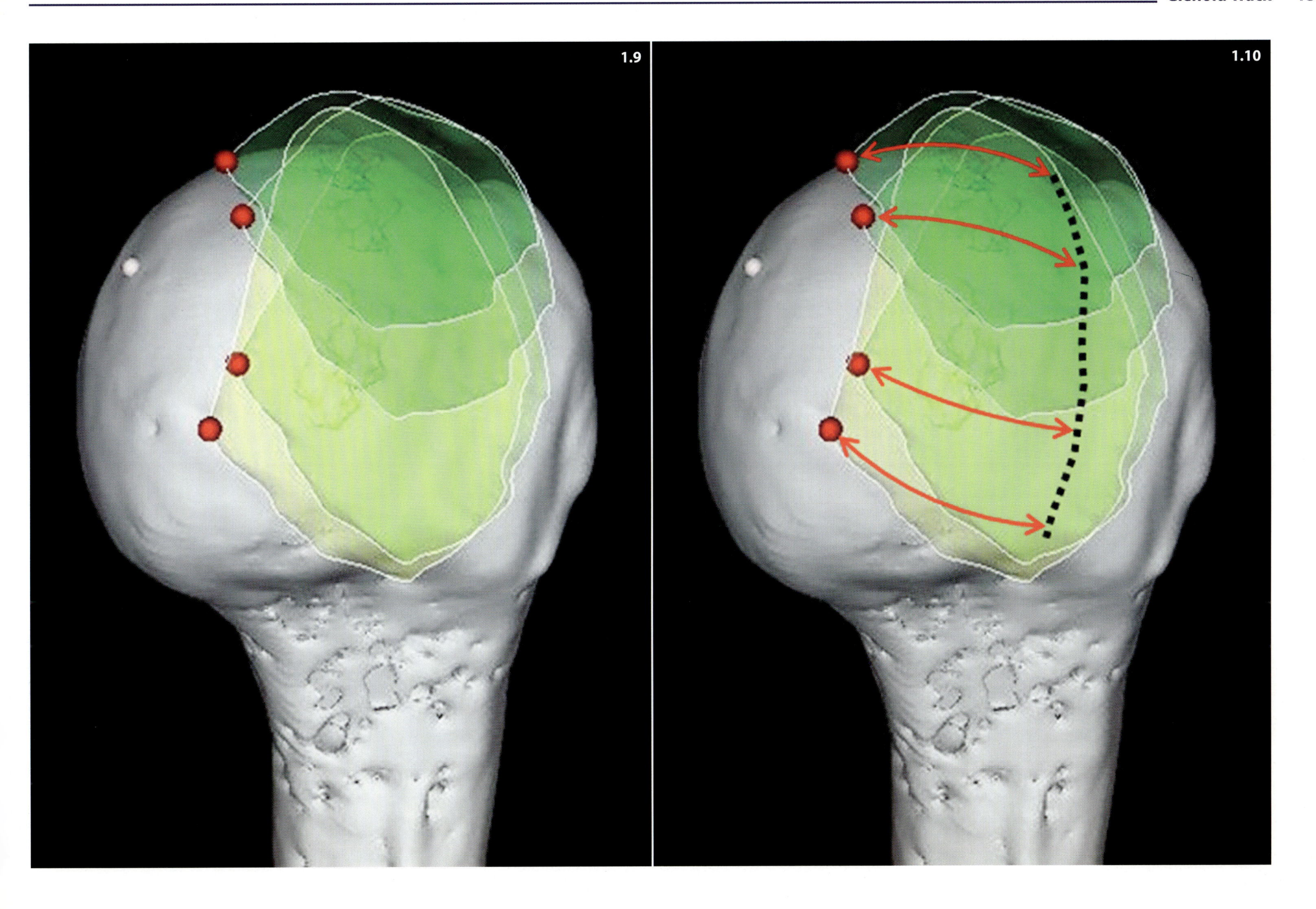
1.9
1.10

References

1. Matsen FA III, Lippitt SB, Bertlesen A et al (2009) Glenohumeral instability. In: Rockwood CA Jr, Matsen FA III, Wirth MA et al (eds) The shoulder, 4th edn, Saunders/Elsevier, Philadelphia, pp 617-770
2. Itoi E, Morrey BF, An KN (2009) Biomechanics of the shoulder. In: Rockwood CA Jr, Matsen FA III, Wirth MA, Lippitt SB (eds) The shoulder, 4th edn. Saunders/Elsevier, Philadelphia, pp 213-265
3. Itoi E (2004) Pathophysiology and treatment of atraumatic instability of the shoulder. J Orthop Sci 9:208-213
4. Rowe CR (1956) Prognosis in dislocations of the shoulder. J Bone Joint Surg Am 38:957-977
5. Itoi E, Hatakeyama Y, Sato T et al (2007) Immobilization in external rotation after shoulder dislocation reduces the risk of recurrence: a randomized controlled trial. J Bone Joint Surg Am 89:2124-2131
6. Nagaraj C, Singh S, Khare GN (2010) A comparative study on effects of position of immobilization on recurrence and quality of life after shoulder dislocation. Read at 11th International Congress on Shoulder and Elbow Surgery, Edinburgh, Sept 5th-8th
7. Finestone A, Milgrom C, Radeva-Petrova DR et al (2009) Bracing in external rotation for traumatic anterior dislocation of the shoulder. J Bone Joint Surg Br 91:918-921
8. Whelan D, Litchfield RB, Boorman RS et al (2008) A randomized evaluation of immobilization in external rotation after primary shoulder dislocation. Read at 75th Annual Meeting, AAOS, San Francisco, March 6
9. Sullivan LG, Bailie R, Weiss N, Miller BS (2007) An evaluation of shoulder external rotation braces. Arthroscopy 23:129-134
10. Jakobsen BW, Johannsen HV, Suder P et al (2007) Primary repair versus conservative treatment of first-time traumatic anterior dislocation of the shoulder: a randomized study with 10-year follow-up. Arthroscopy 23:118-123
11. Bottoni CR, Wilckens JH, DeBerardino TM et al (2002) A prospective, randomized evaluation of arthroscopic stabilization versus nonoperative treatment in patients with acute, traumatic, first-time shoulder dislocations. Am J Sports Med 30:576-580
12. Kirkley A, Werstine R, Ratjek A et al (2005) Prospective randomized clinical trial comparing the effectiveness of immediate arthroscopic stabilization versus immobilization and rehabilitation in first traumatic anterior dislocations of the shoulder: long-term evaluation. Arthroscopy 21:55-63
13. Wheeler JH, Ryan JB, Arciero RA et al (1989) Arthroscopic versus nonoperative treatment of acute shoulder dislocations in young athletes. Arthroscopy 5:213-217
14. Robinson CM, Jenkins PJ, White TO et al (2008) Primary arthroscopic stabilization for a first-time anterior dislocation of the shoulder. A randomized, double-blind trial. J Bone Joint Surg Am 90:708-721
15. Grumet RC, Bach BR Jr, Provencher MT (2010) Arthroscopic stabilization for first-time versus recurrent shoulder instability. Arthroscopy 26:239-248
16. Buss DD, Lynch GP, Meyer CP et al (2004) Nonoperative management for in-season athletes with anterior shoulder instability. Am J Sports Med 32:1430-1433
17. Sugaya H, Moriishi J, Dohi M et al (2003) Glenoid rim morphology in recurrent anterior glenohumeral instability. J Bone Joint Surg Am 85:878-884
18. Calandra JJ, Baker CL, Uribe J (1989) The incidence of Hill-Sachs lesions in initial anterior shoulder dislocations. Arthroscopy 5:254-257
19. Spatschil A, Landsiedl F, Anderl W et al (2006) Posttraumatic anterior-inferior instability of the shoulder: arthroscopic findings and clinical correlations. Arch Orthop Trauma Surg 126:217-222
20. Yiannakopoulos CK, Mataragas E, Antonogiannakis E (2007) A comparison of the spectrum of intra-articular lesions in acute and chronic anterior shoulder instability. Arthroscopy 23:985-990
21. Owens CB, Nelson BJ, Duffey ML et al (2010) Pathoanatomy of first-time, traumatic, anterior glenohumeral subluxation events. J Bone Joint Surg Am 92:1605-1611
22. Rowe CR, Patel D, Southmayd WW (1978) The Bankart procedure: a long-term end-result study. J Bone Joint Surg Am 60:1-16
23. Resch H, Povacz P, Wambacher M et al (1997) Arthroscopic extra-articular Bankart repair for the treatment of recurrent anterior shoulder dislocation. Arthroscopy 13:188-200
24. Savoie FH 3rd, Miller CD, Field LD (1997) Arthroscopic reconstruction of traumatic anterior instability of the shoulder: the Caspari technique. Arthroscopy 13:201-209
25. Saito H, Itoi E, Minagawa H et al (2009) Location of the Hill-Sachs lesion in shoulders with recurrent anterior dislocation. Arch Orthop Trauma Surg 129:1327-1334
26. Rowe CR, Zarins B, Ciullo JV (1984) Recurrent anterior dislocation of the shoulder after surgical repair. Apparent causes of failure and treatment. J Bone Joint Surg Am 66:159-168

27. Bühler M, Gerber C (2002) Shoulder instability related to epileptic seizures. Shoulder Elbow Surg 11:339-344
28. Miniaci A, Berlet G (2001) Recurrent anterior instability following failed surgical repair: allograft reconstruction of large humeral head defects. J Bone Joint Surg Br 83:19-20
29. Hardy P (2003) Bony lesions influence on the result of the arthroscopic treatment of gleno-humeral instability. Symposium: Shoulder instability – limits of arthroscopic surgery: bone deficiency, shrinkage, acute instability. Read at the 5th International Society of Arthroscopy, Knee Surgery and Orthopaedic Sports Medicine Congress, March 10-14; Auckland
30. Yamamoto N, Itoi E, Abe H et al (2007) Contact between the glenoid and the humeral head in abduction, external rotation, and horizontal extension: a new concept of glenoid track. J Shoulder Elbow Surg 16:649-656
31. Omori Y, Yamamoto N, Koishi H et al (2010) Glenoid track in live shoulders using 3D MRI motion analysis. Read at 37th Annual Meeting, Japan Shoulder Society, Sendai, October 8-9
32. Purchase RJ, Wolf EM, Hobgood ER et al (2008) Hill-Sachs "remplissage": an arthroscopic solution for the engaging hill-sachs lesion. Arthroscopy 24:723-726
33. Kazel MD, Sekiya JK, Greene JA et al (2005) Percutaneous correction (humeroplasty) of humeral head defects (Hill-Sachs) associated with anterior shoulder instability: a cadaveric study. Arthroscopy 12:1473-1478
34. Re P, Gallo RA, Richmond JC (2006) Transhumeral head plasty for large Hill-Sachs lesions. Arthroscopy 22:e1-e4
35. Connolly JF (1972) Humeral head defects associated with shoulder dislocations – their diagnostic and surgical significance. Instr Course Lect 21:42-54
36. Weber BG, Simpson LA, Hardegger F (1984) Rotational humeral osteotomy for recurrent anterior dislocation of the shoulder associated with a large Hill-Sachs lesion. J Bone Joint Surg Am 66: 1443-1450
37. Regan WD Jr, Webster-Bogaert S, Hawkins RJ et al (1989) Comparative functional analysis of the Bristow, Magnuson-Stack, and Putti-Platt procedures for recurrent dislocation of the shoulder. Am J Sports Med 17:42-48
38. Burkhart SS, De Beer JF (2000) Traumatic glenohumeral bone defects and their relationship to failure of arthroscopic Bankart repairs: significance of the inverted-pear glenoid and the humeral engaging Hill-Sachs lesion. Arthroscopy 16:677-694

Chapter 2 – Shoulder Instability: Glenoid and Humeral-head Bone Defect

Paolo Baudi, Paolo Righi, Eugenio Rossi Urtoler and Giuseppe Milano

2.1 Introduction

Glenohumeral bone loss is one of the most important factors responsible for failure and recurrence after a shoulder arthroscopic instability repair. A high percentage of patients with traumatic, recurrent anterior instability have some level of glenohumeral bone loss. It is necessary to recognize the amount of bone loss preoperatively in order to determine successful management strategies. Standard radiographs may be inadequate for detecting the extent of glenoid and humeral-head bone loss.

Glenoid fractures and bony Bankart should be distinguished from attritional glenoid bone loss in which the injured portion of glenoid bone has resorbed. Two- and three-dimensional computed tomography (CT) are useful for quantitative assessment of glenoid bone loss and can be done using different methods: the true circle method on 2D CT (Pico method) appears most reliable and could be theoretically used without comparison.

Three-dimensional CT is an accurate method for sizing and localizing osteochondral lesions of the humeral head and can be used for grading Hill-Sachs lesions. CT scan with 3D reconstruction is necessary if any bone loss is visible on X-ray or magnetic resonance imaging (MRI). Location is more important than size: Hill-Sachs lesions will only "engage" if they extend medially over medial margin of glenoid rim.

In recent years, many authors focused on the importance of glenoid and humeral bone defects associated with anterior glenohumeral instability. Biomechanical studies showed that glenoid and humeral bone defects can affect normal shoulder kinematics by changing glenohumeral contact forces and reducing resistance to dislocation. Further, clinical studies reported a significant incidence of bony Bankart lesion and Hill-Sachs lesion after first dislocation, a high percentage of glenoid bone loss in chronic instability, and a significant correlation between the amount of glenohumeral bone loss and recurrence rate of instability after surgical treatment. For these reasons, detection and quantification of glenoid and humeral bone defects have implications for treatment choice, and most recent guidelines on the treatment of anterior glenohumeral instability recommend open procedures by bone reconstruction or augmentation when major glenoid and/or humeral bone loss is present.

It is imperative that adequate radiographic imaging be included in workup of patients with recurrent shoulder instability. Glenoid bone loss is the likely number one reason shoulder instability surgery fails. However, with adequate preoperative evaluation of glenoid and humeral-head bone defects, the surgeon may be able to present a more informed decision to the patient regarding overall management and risk of recurrence.

2.2 Glenoid-bone Defect

Glenoid-bone defect and recurrence after stabilization surgery has been reported by several authors. In 1961, Rowe [1] reported an incidence of recurrent dislocation that rose from 6% to 62% if glenoid bone defect was present. In 2000, Burkhart and De Beer [2] analyzed 194 patients operated by the two authors using the same method (suture anchor technique) and selected 21 recurrences. The incidence of recurrence in the group without deficit was 4% and in the group with bone defect 67%, particularly if the patients participated in contact sports. The glenoid with bone defect was defined as an inverted pear because it appears similar to a pear rotated 180°. Tauber and Resh [3] reviewed 41 patients who had had recurrence of instability and identified a bone deficit of the glenoid rim in 56% of cases, capsular injury in 27%, and recurrence of Bankart in 17%. In 2003, Lim [4] presented a study conducted on 20 patients with glenoid defect and 20 without bone defect who had undergone open surgery involving Bankart capsule-ligament reinsertion and observed a significant deficit in rotation and a 5% incidence of recurrence (vs 0%) in patients with bone defect.

Once the relationship between recurrence and bone defect has been established, an anatomopathologic and radiologic classification of the lesion of the glenoid is necessary. In 1998, Bigliani et al. [5] first coined the term bony Bankart to indicate the presence in cases of instability of an anteroinferior bone fragment with preserved insertion of the inferior glenohumeral ligament (Bigliani type 1). He also determined a type 2 in which the fragment had poorly consolidated and the relationship with the ligament complex was no longer recognizable. Finally, he introduced the concept of glenoid bone defect, classifying an erosion that was <25% (type 3A) and one that was >25% (type 3B) of the total glenoid surface. In type B cases, he believed it was necessary to proceed with bone graft. Edwards Walchet al. [6] classified glenoid bone loss into three forms after radiologic examination [X-ray in the anteroposterior (AP) and Bernageau views]: bony Bankart, that is, fracture with fragment still visible; bone loss with loss of anteroinferior angle without visible fragment (cliff sign); bone loss with rounding compression of the glenoid rim (blunted angle). It is important to establish the frequency of bone defect in acute glenohumeral dislocation (first episode) and in chronic instability. Edwards et al. [6] reported a 90% of glenoid bone lesion in 160 chronic unstable shoulders diagnosed by radiologic examination alone (AP and Bernageau profile). Griffith et al. [7] demonstrated the presence of anteroinferior bone defects of the glenoid in 90% of shoulders affected with instability compared with 4% in healthy contralateral shoulders. Sugaya et al. [8] studied 100 unstable shoulders with CT in 3D and monitored arthroscopically, to determine only 10% normal shoulders, 40% erosion-compression of the glenoid rim, and 50% bony Bankart. No consensus exists as to what constitutes severe glenoid bone loss, and it is important to define the critical entity of the bone defect in addition to planning bone-graft surgery. Bigliani et al. [5] suggested a 25% reduction in glenoid width as a reasonable cut off. In their experimental study, Itoi et al. [9, 10] found that a lesion of 21% of the glenoid length decreased by 50% the intrinsic stability provided by the glenoid and showed how this amount of bone defect corresponded to a deficit of 18% in the West Point X-ray examination and to a loss of 50% of glenoid depth on CT slice through the lower one fourth. A potential limitation of this latter study is that defects were created on the anteroinferior margin of the glenoid, whereas recently, studies indicate that, in recurrent dislocation, principal bone loss occurs anteriorly rather than anteroinferiorly. Burkhart and De Beer [11] in 2002 and Burkhart and Lo in 2004 [12] attempted to determine the entity of a critical glenoid bone loss and illustrated an arthroscopic method. This critical anterior defect was 8.6 mm ± 2.2 mm, corresponding to a mean loss of 36% of depth of the inferior glenoid able to create an image like an inverted pear.

Different ways to identify and measure the size of a glenoid bone defect have been described in the literature using preoperative imaging techniques or intraoperative arthroscopic methods [6, 11, 13–17]. Arthroscopic measurement is based on the glenoid bare spot as landmark of the center of the inferior glenoid [11, 18]. Quantification of the defect is assessed by calculating the difference between posterior and anterior radii of the inferior glenoid and the ratio between this difference and the diameter of the intact glenoid (equal to posterior radius × 2) [11]. However, some anatomical studies [19–21] showed that the inferior glenoid has the shape of a true circle, but the bare spot is not exactly in the center. Moreover, Provencher et al. [22] recently observed in a cadaver study that bone-loss measurement with the bare spot method overestimates the area of the missing glenoid, especially for small defects. Finally, it must be considered that the presence and size of a glenoid defect can influence the choice of surgical procedure, so that a preoperative assessment would be more valuable.

Some authors [5, 6, 17] focused on the use of specific radiographic views (Figs. 2.1 and 2.2) (i.e., true AP, Stryker notch, West Point and Bernageau view) to diagnose a glenoid defect in anterior shoulder instability, but none of these methods was tested for reliability and accuracy in quantifying bone loss.

Fig. 2.1. True anteroposterior X-ray

Fig. 2.2. Bernageau view

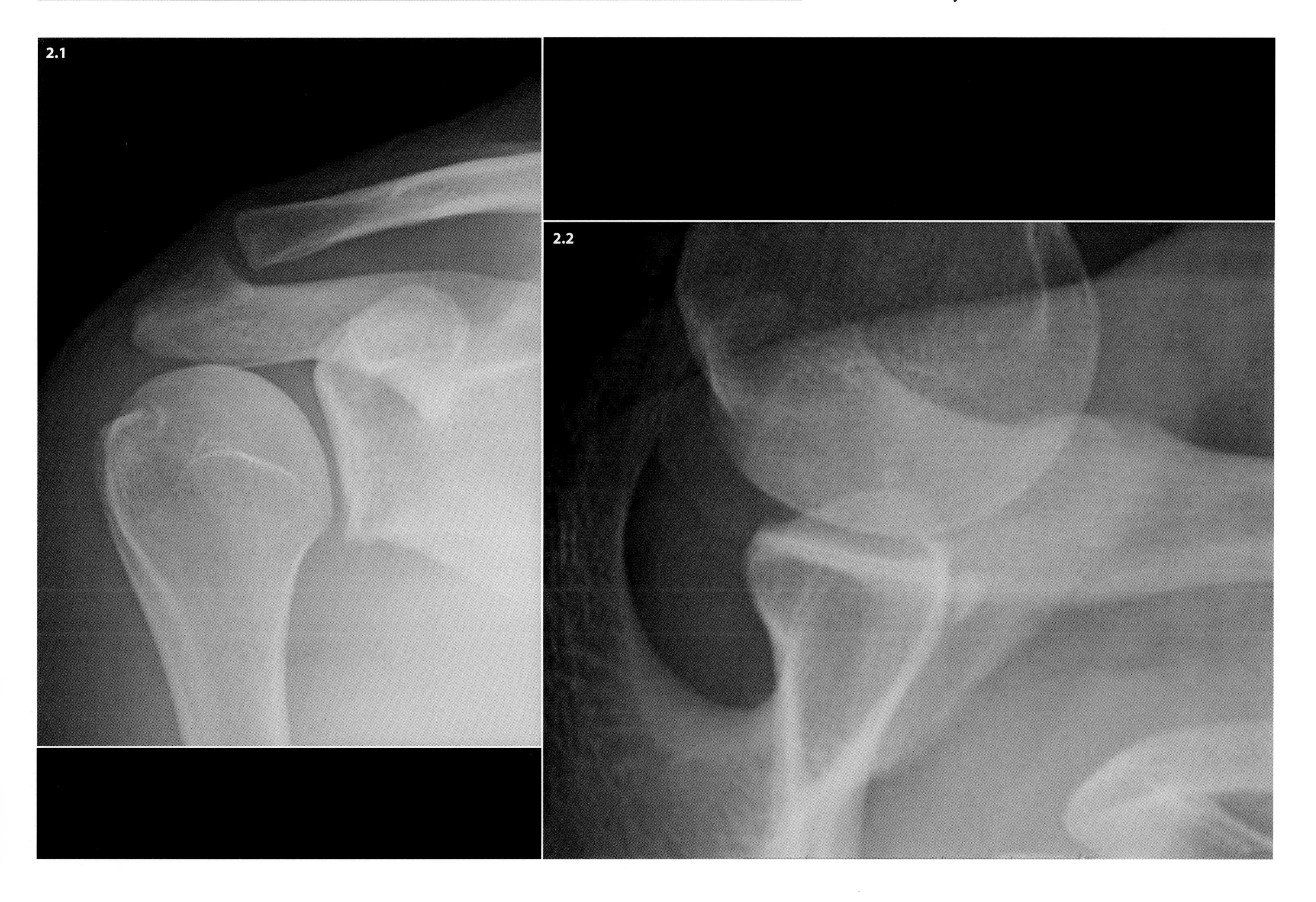
2.1
2.2

MRI is considered as the first option for evaluating soft tissue injuries in shoulder instability (Fig. 2.3); however, few studies recognize its utility in diagnosing glenoid bone defects [13, 23, 24]. Conversely, many authors [14, 16, 25–31] report using computed tomography (CT), with both the 3D volume-rendered technique (VRT) (Fig. 2.4) and 2D multiplanar reformation (MPR) scans as the modalities of choice to detect bony abnormalities in glenohumeral instability. Griffith et al. [14] described a method for quantification of a glenoid defect using MPR CT images based on the ratio between the maximum width of the affected glenoid and that of the contralateral healthy glenoid. Chuang et al. [26] recently proposed a method for measuring glenoid bone defect on 3D CT images similar to that by Griffith et al. [14]. They described the glenoid index as the ratio between the width of the injured glenoid and preinjury glenoid width (similar to that of the contralateral healthy shoulder). Both methods were validated for accuracy using the arthroscopic measurement as reference technique [26, 31]; however, accuracy of arthroscopic measurement has not been assessed in previous studies. Barchilon et al. [25] reported on a trigonometric method to measure glenoid defect on CT scans with and without 3D reconstruction using the ratio between defect depth and inferior glenoid radius, but they did not validated the method.

The circle method is an alternative technique for evaluating glenoid bone defect in preoperative imaging studies. It is based on the observation that the inferior part of the glenoid has the shape of a true circle, which can be drawn on the sagittal en face view of the glenoid [16, 19, 32]. The advantage of this method is direct measurement on the affected glenoid without comparison with the contralateral healthy glenoid. The circle method was first proposed using 3D CT images, shown to be very accurate [13]. Sugaya et al. [8] analyzed glenoid bone defects on 3D CT images and found an abnormal configuration of the anterior glenoid in 90% of patients with recurrent unilateral anterior shoulder instability; however, the method was not validated for reliability. Huysmans et al. [19] used the circle method proposed by Sugaya et al. [8] on 14 cadaver shoulders to validate 3D CT scans and MRI to quantify the glenoid bone defect. Both methods showed a very good intraobserver and interobserver reliability; however, limited number of samples analyzed (14 glenoids) makes results of the study rather inconclusive.

Baudi et al. [33] developed a CT method, named Pico (in honor of the Italian philosopher Pico della Mirandola; Mirandola 1463 – Florence 1494) to detect and measure glenoid bone defects in terms of surface area and percentage by processing images in MPR. The Pico method by Baudi et al. [33] combines the advantages of the circle method (direct measurement of the missing area of the glenoid) with those of the MPR technique (neither 3D reconstructions nor subtraction images are required). Furthermore, MPR allows a real measurement of the size of the missing bone (length and width), which can be useful when a bone grafting procedure is planned to restore glenoid anatomy. This information cannot be obtained with VRT, where measurements are expressed in pixels and therefore the magnitude of bone loss can only be calculated as a percentage of the intact glenoid. Finally, VRT implies a greater risk of artefacts than does the MPR technique, which can impair interpretation of the exam.

Fig. 2.3. Magnetic resonance imaging sagittal view

Fig. 2.4. Bony Bankart lesion in 3D volume-rendered technique

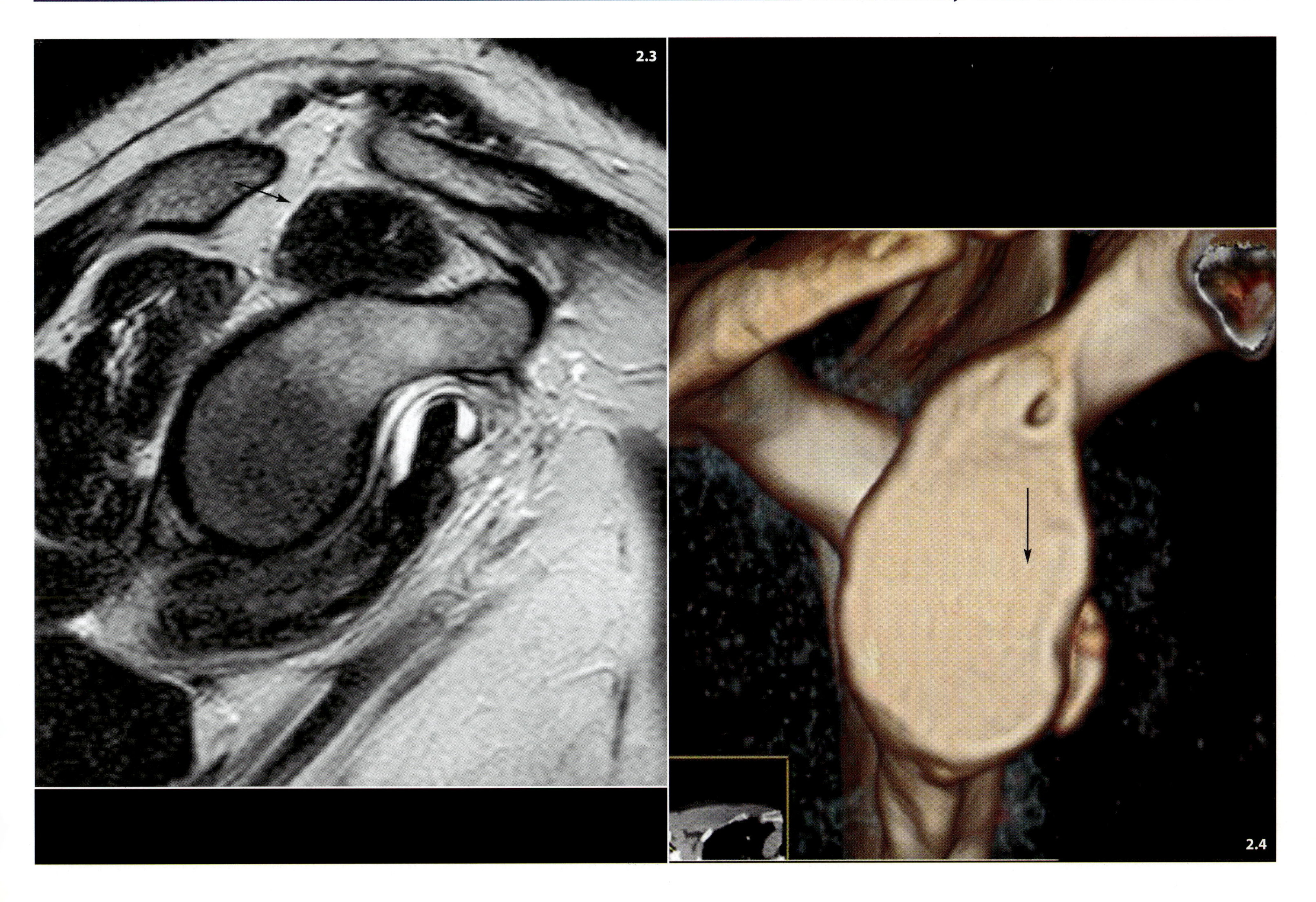
2.3
2.4

2.2.1 CT Examination Technique

All patients underwent a CT scan of both shoulders at the same time with a spiral double-slice CT (e.g., LightSpeed Pro16; GE Healthcare) that used filter for bone, 1.25-mm slice thickness with slice advancement of 0.6 mm, 200–300 mA, 120 kV, FOV 30 cm, matrix 512 × 512 pixels. The scanning plane extended from the acromion-clavicular joint to just below the glenoid. Images were processed on a CT workstation (ADW 4.2) in MPR according to oblique sagittal planes, maintaining working axes parallel to the glenoid surface, to obtain oblique sagittal images of the glenoid articular surface (en face view). On this frontal image of the healthy glenoid, a circumferential area was drawn on the inferior part of the glenoid using the digital analysis software of the workstation. The best-fitting circle on the inferior glenoid was used by selecting the outer cortex of the inferior glenoid (from 3 to 9 o'clock) as landmark. Therefore, an identical circumference was drawn on the affected glenoid, and the area of the circle (A) and the missing part of that circle (D) were measured (mm^2) (Fig. 2.5). The size of the defect was expressed as percentage of the entire circle, according to the following formula:

$$\text{Surface D} / \text{Surface A} \times 100$$

Baudi et al. [33] reported a preliminary study on the Pico method on 46 patients with shoulder instability and found a glenoid defect in 54% cases. In a complete study on 115 patients presented during an instructional course of the Upper Extremity Committee of the European Society of Sports Traumatology Knee Surgery and Arthroscopy (ESSKA) [34], a glenoid bone defect was reported for 65% of patients and a Hill-Sachs lesion in 80%. Our study indicates that glenoid bone loss in recurrent anterior dislocation probably takes three distinct forms: the first is the anterior or anteroinferior glenoid rim fracture (bony Bankart) that results from avulsion of the glenohumeral ligament complex during dislocation (Fig. 2.6). The second is anterior bone loss that most likely results from a compressive injury, as the dislocated humerus subsequently impacts

Fig. 2.5. Pico method with 2D multiplanar reformation

Fig. 2.6. Pico method for bony Bankart lesion

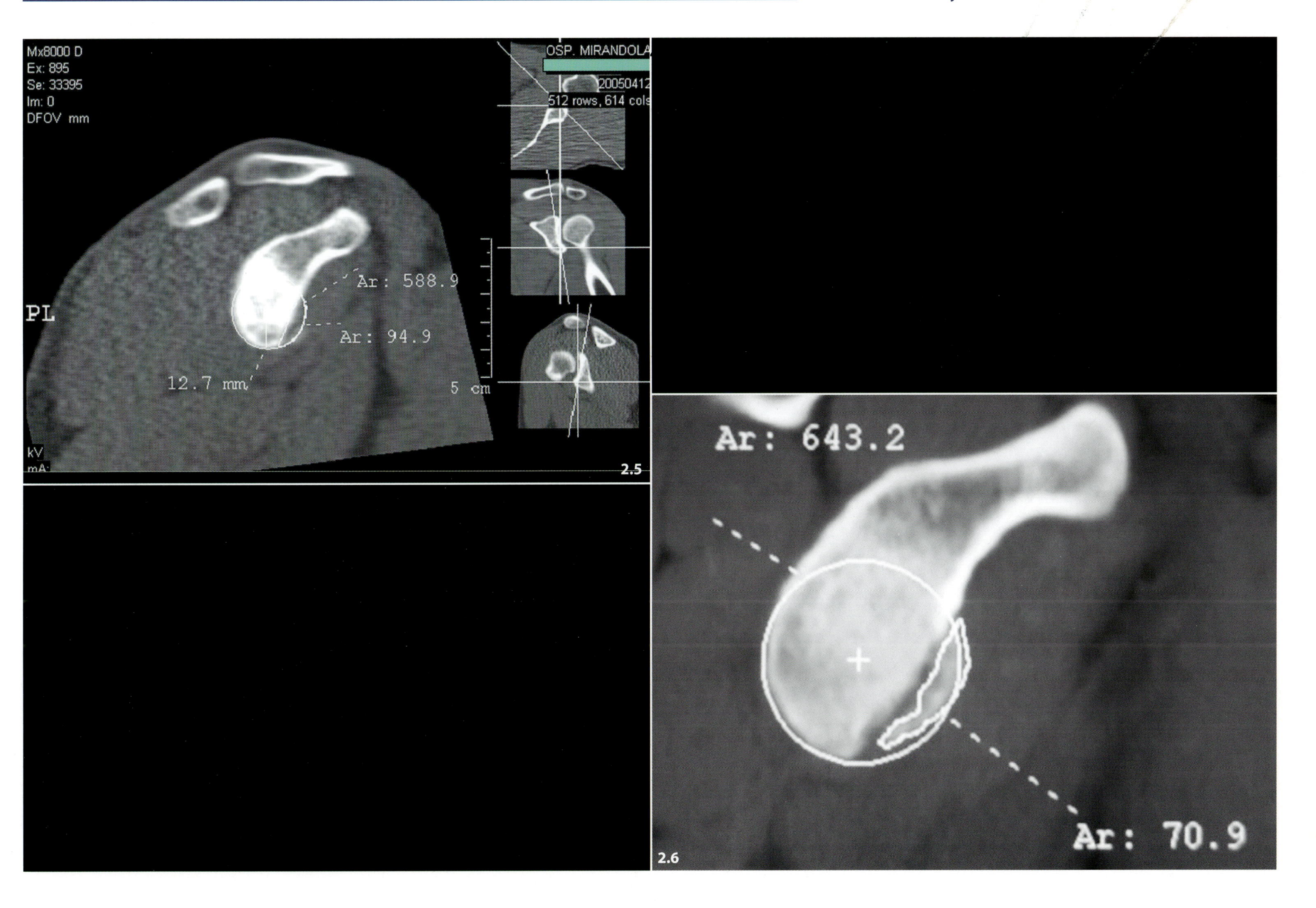
Mx8000 D
Ex: 895
Se: 33395
Im: 0
DFOV mm
OSP. MIRANDOLA
20050412
512 rows, 614 cols
Ar: 588.9
PL
Ar: 94.9
12.7 mm
5 cm
kV
mA
2.5
Ar: 643.2
Ar: 70.9
2.6

the anterior glenoid rim. In this type of lesion, called straight pear, it is possible to define a straight lane from 2 o'clock to 5 o'clock with a range of glenoid bone defect between 5% and 15%, and this type of lesion is very frequently from 55% to 65 % [30, 34] (Fig. 2.7). The last type of lesion is an anteroinferior defect that results from a high-energy trauma or a neglected glenoid fracture, with an oblique lane from 3 o'clock to 6 o'clock and a defect >20% but with a low frequency from 5% to 10% [30, 34].

A recent study was published to confirm a very good intraobserver and interobserver reliability of the Pico CT method to quantify glenoid bone defect in anterior glenohumeral instability [35]. This study enlisted 40 patients (35 men and five women) with unilateral anterior shoulder instability with at least one episode of dislocation. The inferior part of a normal glenoid perfectly fitted the drawn circle at all measurements in 36 cases (90%). Mean missing part of the circle in the remaining four cases was 0.32% for the first observer (average of three measurements) and 0.48% for the second observer. Missing part of the circle in normal glenoids did not exceed 1%. Mean values [± standard deviation (SD)] of glenoid-bone defects were considered for the first measurement of the first observer, the average of the three measurements of the first observer, and the single measurement of the second observer. Mean glenoid-bone defect was 5.1 ± 6.8% (range 0–33%) for first measurement of the first observer, 4.8 ± 6.4% (range 0–33%) for average measurement of the first observer, and 4.5 ± 6.3% (range 0–34.5%) for the single measurement of the second observer.

Analysis of intraobserver reliability showed intraclass correlation coefficient (ICC) values of 0.94 [95% confidence interval (CI) = 0.89–0.96] for single measurement and 0.98 (95% CI = 0.96–0.99) for average measurement. Standard error of mean (SEM) was 1.1% for single measurement and 1.0% for average measurement. Analysis of interobserver reliability showed ICC values of 0.90 (95% CI = 0.82–0.95) for single measurement and 0.95 (95% CI = 0.90–0.97) for average measurement. SEM was 1.0% both for single and average measurements.

The Pico method appears to be more reliable than measurement of maximum glenoid width. The method is based on the circle of the inferior glenoid and could be theoretically used without comparison with the contralateral shoulder, which is different from the method by Griffith et al. [14]. The Pico method can be used even in recurrent instability after arthroscopic treatment (stabilization) with metallic or adsorbable anchors (Fig. 2.8).

Fig. 2.7. Pico method for attritional glenoid-bone loss

Fig. 2.8. Pico method in recurrent dislocation after arthroscopic stabilization

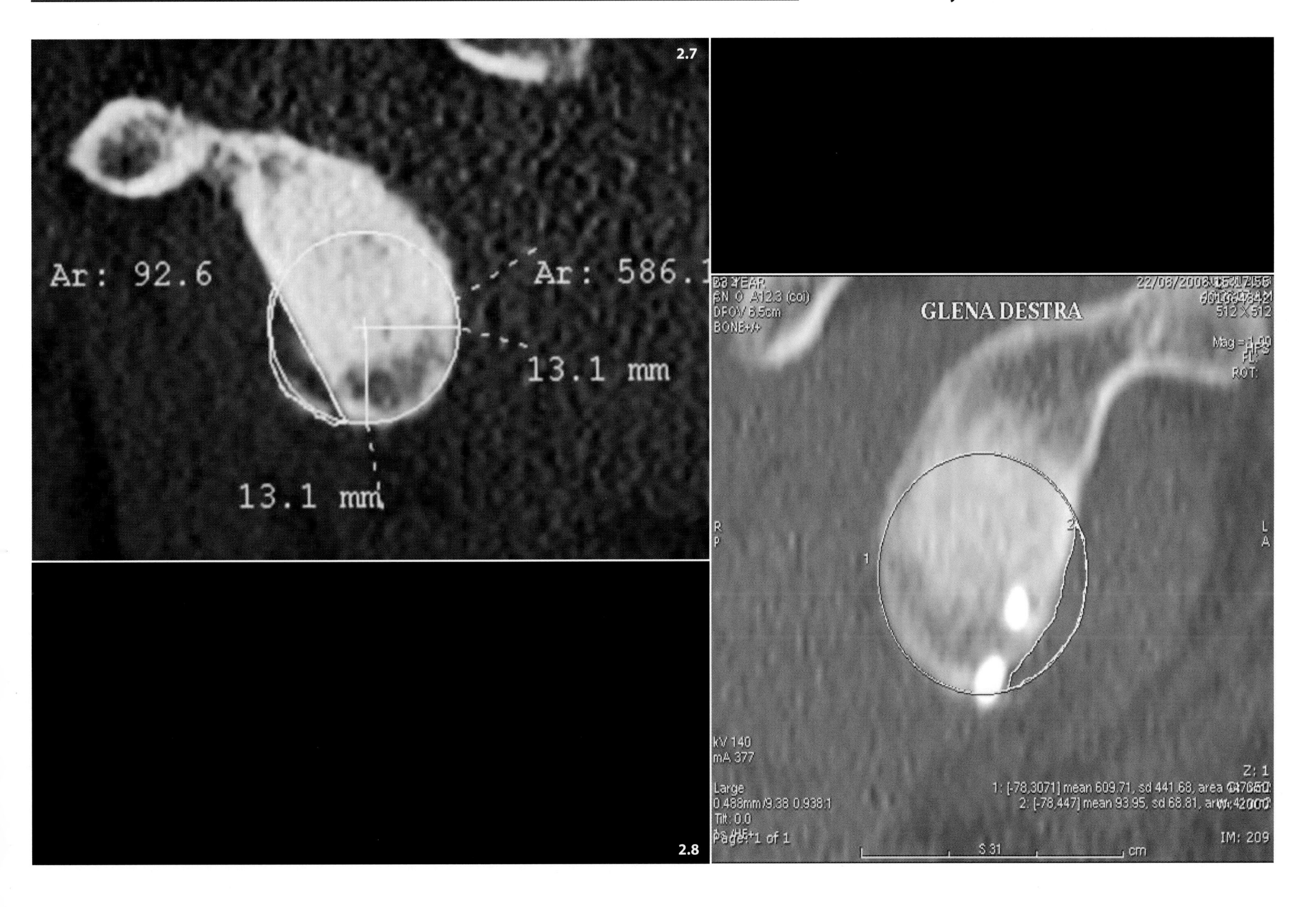
2.7
Ar: 92.6
Ar: 586.
13.1 mm
13.1 mm
2.8
GLENA DESTRA
DFOV 6.5cm
512 X 512
kV 140
mA 377
Large
Tilt: 0.0
R
P
L
A
1
2
Z: 1
IM: 209
cm

2.3 Humeral Bone Loss

As with the glenoid, the humeral head may also demonstrate a high percentage of osseous pathology after traumatic anterior dislocation. Osteochondral defects in the humeral head, often referred to as Hill-Sachs lesions, are commonly found on the posterolateral region where the soft base of the humeral head impacts against the anterior glenoid rim. They are caused by a compression fracture that forms when the humeral head is displaced anteriorly, inferiorly, and medially during traumatic dislocation. Hill-Sachs lesions can be formed during the initial or subsequent episode of anterior shoulder dislocation. It has been reported that almost half of initial anterior shoulder dislocations are accompanied by a Hill-Sachs lesion [36]. Such osteochondral lesions often play a fundamental role in recurrent shoulder instability by decreasing the humeral head's contribution to passive stability. When the arm abducts and externally rotates, the Hill-Sachs lesion comes into contact with the anterior glenoid rim, thereby causing the rim to drop into and engage the Hill-Sachs lesion [37]. Hill-Sachs lesions can be detected and quantified using a variety of imaging techniques, including radiography, MRI, and MR arthrography. Humeral-head bone loss can also be assessed using an AP view with internal rotation and the Stryker-notch view, but the best radiographic view for identifying humeral-head bone loss after traumatic anterior dislocation – namely, Hill-Sachs lesions – is the Stryker-notch view. In a prospective study of 27 shoulders with recurrent anterior dislocation, Rozing et al. found the Stryker-notch view to adequately demonstrate Hill-Sachs lesions in 92.6% of shoulders [38]. A study by Workman et al. retrospectively compared diagnostic interpretations of plain film radiography, arthroscopy, and MRI [39]. The authors concluded that MRI was the most reliable method for Hill-Sachs lesion documentation and superior to arthroscopy. When two or three imaging modalities were utilized for assigning a final diagnosis of Hill-Sachs lesion, MRI demonstrated sensitivity of 97%, specificity of 91%, and accuracy of 94%. One reason Hill-Sachs lesions are not usually missed on MRI is that they are frequently accompanied by abnormal signal intensity within the marrow of the humeral head – a sign of bony contusion related to the mechanism of injury. Rowe et al. [40] graded Hill-Sachs lesions based on dimensions measured intraoperatively during reoperations for failed surgical treatment of recurrent anterior dislocations. To characterize osseous defects, the length and depth on preoperative imaging are measured. Moderate lesions are classified as those between 0.5 and 1cm deep and 2 and 4 cm long. Lesions with dimensions larger than these are considered severe, whereas smaller lesions are classified as mild. Quantifying the size of humeral-head lesions is crucial to preoperative planning, and 3D CT is the most accurate method to size and localize the Hill-Sachs lesion (Fig. 2.9). Recently, some authors have used clinical data to conclude that Bankart repair is ineffective in situations where the Hill-Sachs lesion depth is >16% of the humeral-head diameter or volume is >1,000 mm^3 [41].

In addition to determining the amount bone loss associated with a Hill-Sachs lesion, location on the humeral head must also be assessed. According to Yamamoto et al. [42], the glenoid track is a zone of contact between articular surfaces of the humeral head and glenoid as the arm is ranged through varying degrees of abduction. As long as the Hill-Sachs lesion remains within the glenoid track, there is no chance of it overriding the glenoid rim and causing instability or anterior dislocation. The lesion only has a chance of engaging if it extends medially over the medial margin of the glenoid track (Fig. 2.10). Thus, lesion location relative to the glenoid track is more important than lesion size [42].

2.4 Conclusion

In conclusion, it is imperative to determine precisely the amount of glenoid bone loss and location of the Hill-Sachs lesion in order to correlate them with the most important risk factors for arthroscopic shoulder stabilization (age; sex; type of sport/work). The Pico method is useful, reliable, and accurate for assessing glenoid-bone defect, and 3D CT is necessary to determine the size and location of a Hill-Sachs lesion.

Fig. 2.9. Hill-Sachs lesion on 3D computed tomography reconstruction

Fig. 2.10. Hill-Sachs lesion extended medially over the medial margin of glenoid track

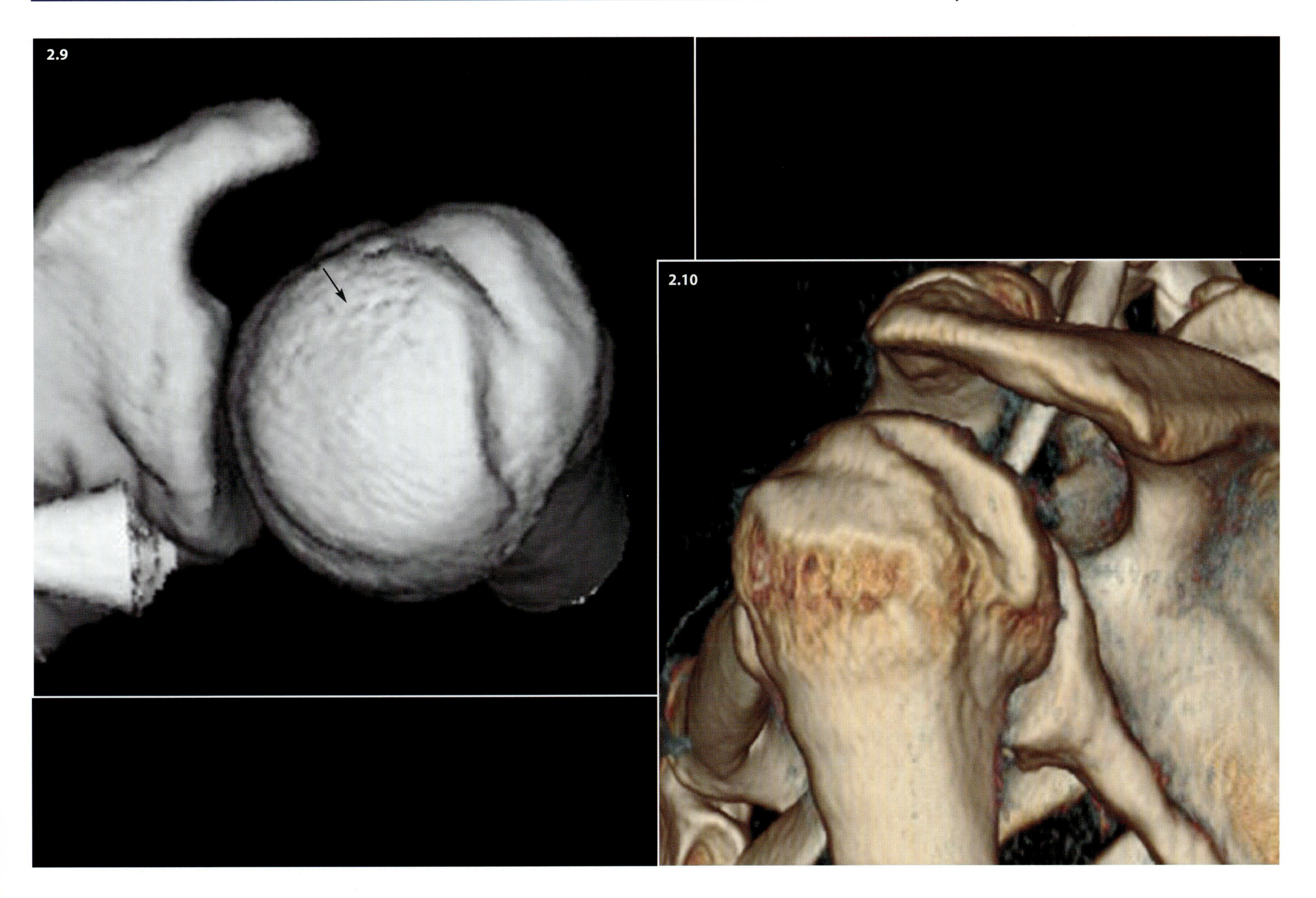
2.9
2.10

References

1. Rowe CR (1961) Factors related to recurrences of anterior dislocation of the shoulder. Clin Orthop 20:40-48
2. Burkhart SS De Beer JF (2002) Traumatic glenohumeral bone defects and their relationship to failure of arthroscopic Bankart repairs: significance of the inverted-pear glenoid and the humeral engaging Hill-Sachs lesion. Arthroscopy 16:677-694
3. Tauber M, Resch H (2004) Reason for failure after surgical repair of anterior shoulder instability. J Shoulder Elbow Surg 13:279-285
4. Lim CT Rhee YG SECEC (2003) Abstract Book Oral 7: shoulder instability, pp 119
5. Bigliani LU, Newton PM, Steinmann SP et al (1998) Glenoid rim lesions associated with recurrent anterior dislocation of the shoulder. Am J Sports Med 26:41-45
6. Edwards TB, Boulahia A, Walch G (2003) Radiographic analysis of bone defects in chronic anterior shoulder instability. Arthroscopy 19:732-739
7. Griffith JF, Antonio GE, Tong CW, Ming CK (2003) Anterior shoulder dislocation: quantification of glenoid bone loss with CT. AJR Am J Roentgenol 180:1423-1430
8. Sugaya H, Moriishi J, Dohi M (2003) Glenoid rim morphology in recurrent anterior glenohumeral instability. J Bone Joint Surg Am 85:878-884
9. Itoi E, Lee SB, Berglund LJ et al (2000) The effect of a glenoid defect on anteroinferior stability of the shoulder after Bankart repair: a cadaveric study. J Bone Joint Surg Am 82:35-46
10. Itoi E, Lee SB, Amrami KK et al (2003) Quantitative assessment of classic anteroinferior bony Bankart lesions by radiography and computed tomography. Am J Sports Med 31:112-118
11. Burkhart SS De Beer JF (2002) Quantifying glenoid bone loss arthroscopically in shoulder instability. Arthroscopy 18:488-491
12. Burkhart SS, Lo IK (2004) The inverted pear glenoid: an indicator of significant glenoid bone loss. Arthroscopy 20:169-174
13. Huijsmans PE, Haen PS, Kidd M et al (2007) Quantification of a glenoid defect with three-dimensional computed tomography and magnetic resonance imaging: a cadaveric study. J Shoulder Elbow Surg 16:803-809
14. Griffith JF, Antonio GE, Tong CW, Ming CK (2003) Anterior shoulder dislocation: quantification of glenoid bone loss with CT. AJR Am J Roentgenol 180:1423-1430
15. Itoi E, Lee SB, Amrami KK et al (2003) Quantitative assessment of classic anteroinferior bony Bankart lesions by radiography and computed tomography. Am J Sports Med 31:112-118
16. Sugaya H, Moriishi J, Dohi M et al (2003) Glenoid rim morphology in recurrent anterior glenohumeral instability. J Bone Joint Surg Am 85:878-884
17. Pavlov H, Warren RF, Weiss CB Jr (1985) The roentgenographic evaluation of anterior shoulder instability. Clin Orthop Rel Res 194:153-158
18. De Wilde LF, Berghs BM, Audenaert E et al (2004) About the variability of the shape of the glenoid cavity. Surg Radiol Anat 26:54-59
19. Huysmans PE, Haen PS, Kidd M et al (2006) The shape of the inferior part of the glenoid: a cadaveric study. J Shoulder Elbow Surg 15:759-763
20. Kralinger F, Aigner F, Longato S et al (2006) Is the bare spot a consistent landmark for shoulder arthroscopy? A study of 20 embalmed glenoids with 3-dimensional computed tomographic reconstruction. Arthroscopy 22:428-432
21. Aigner F, Longato S, Fritsch H, Kralinger F (2004) Anatomical considerations regarding the "bare spot" of the glenoid cavity. Surg Radiol Anat 26:308-311
22. Provencher MT, Detterline AJ, Ghodadra N et al (2008) Measurement of glenoid bone loss: a comparison of measurement error between 45 degrees and 0 degrees bone loss models and with different posterior arthroscopy portal locations. Am J Sports Med 36:1132-1138
23. Willemsen UF, Wiedemann E, Brunner U et al (1998) Prospective evaluation of MR arthrography performed with high-volume intraarticular saline enhancement in patients with recurrent anterior dislocations of the shoulder. AJR Am J Roentgenol 170:79-84
24. Stoller D, Shellock FG, Crues JV (1996) MRI of the shoulder: a rational approach to the reporting of findings. J Magn Reson Imaging 6:268-270
25. Barchilon VS, Kotz E, Barchilon Ben-Av M et al (2008) A simple method for quantitative evaluation of the missing area of the anterior glenoid in anterior instability of the glenohumeral joint. Skeletal Radiol 37:731-736
26. Chuang TY, Adams CR, Burkhart SS (2008) Use of preoperative three-dimensional computed tomography to quantify glenoid bone loss in shoulder instability. Arthroscopy 24:376-382
27. Saito H, Itoi E, Sugaya H et al (2005) Location of the glenoid defect in shoulders with recurrent anterior dislocation. Am J Sports Med 33:889-893

28. Stevens KJ, Preston BJ, Wallace WA, Kerslake RW (1999) CT and 3D reconstructions of shoulders with anterior glenohumeral instability. Clin Anat 12:326-336
29. Diederichs G, Seim H, Meyer H et al (2008) CT-based patient-specific modeling of glenoid rim defects: a feasibility study. AJR Am J Roentgenol 191:1406-1411
30. Griffith JF, Antonio GE, Yung PS et al (2008) Prevalence, pattern, and spectrum of glenoid bone loss in anterior shoulder dislocation: CT analysis of 218 patients. AJR Am J Roentgenol 190:1247-1254
31. Griffith JF, Yung PS, Antonio GE (2007) CT compared with arthroscopy in quantifying glenoid bone loss. AJR Am J Roentgenol 189:1490-1493
32. Jeske HC, Oberthaler M, Klingensmith M et al (2009) Normal glenoid rim anatomy and the reliability of shoulder instability measurements based on intrasite correlation. Surg Radiol Anat 31:623-625
33. Baudi P, Righi P, Bolognesi D et al (2005) How to identify and calculate glenoid bone deficit. Chir Organi Mov 90:145-152
34. Baudi P (2008) Instructional Course of ESSKA Upper Extremity Committee: how to manage bone defects in shoulder instability. In: 13th ESSKA 2000 Congress, 2008 Porto/Portugal
35. Magarelli N, Milano G, Sergio P et al (2009) Intra-observer and inter-observer reliability of the 'Pico' computed tomography method for quantification of glenoid bone defect in anterior shoulder instability. Skeletal Radiol 38:1071-1075
36. Calandra JJ, Baker CL, Uribe J (1989) The incidence of Hill-Sachs lesions in initial anterior shoulder dislocations. Arthroscopy 5:254-247
37. Burkhart SS, Danaceau SM (2000) Articular length mismatch as a cause of failed Bankart repair. Arthroscopy 16:740-744
38. Rozing PM, de Bakker HM, Obermann WR (1986) Radiographic views in recurrent anterior shoulder dislocation. Comparison of six methods for identification of typical lesions. Acta Orthop Scand 57:328-330
39. Workman TL, Burkhard TK, Resnick D et al. (1992) Hill-Sachs lesion: comparison of detection with MR imaging, radiography, and arthroscopy. Radiology 185:847-852
40. Rowe CR, Zarins B, Ciullo, JV (1984) Recurrent anterior dislocation of the shoulder after surgical repair. Apparent causes of failure and treatment. J Bone Joint Surg Am 66: 159-168
41. Hardy P (2003) Bony lesions influence on the result of the arthroscopic treatment of gleno-humeral instability. Symposium: Shoulder instability-limits of arthroscopic surgery: bone deficiency, shrinkage, acute instability. In: 5th International Society of Arthroscopy, Knee Surgery and Orthopaedic Sports Medicine Congress. Auckland
42. Yamamoto N, Itoi E, Abe H et al (2007) Contact between the glenoid and the humeral head in abduction, external rotation, and horizontal extension: a new concept of glenoid track. J Shoulder Elbow Surg 16:649-656

Chapter 3 – Latarjet Procedure: the Miniplate Surgical Technique

Giovanni Di Giacomo, Alberto Costantini, Andrea De Vita and Nicola de Gasperis

3.1 Introduction

The Latarjet procedure [1], first described in 1958 and used to address anteroinferior shoulder instability, involves using coracoid transfer to stabilize the shoulder by the static action of the transferred bone block and by the dynamic action of the attached conjoined tendon sling (short head of biceps and coracobrachialis). There are different effects by which to achieve shoulder stability with the Latarjet procedure:

- bone effect: bone graft can prevent engagement of a humeral bone lesion because the graft extends the glenoid arch to such a degree that the shoulder cannot externally rotate far enough to engage the Hill-Sachs lesion over the front of the graft [2];
- muscle effect: transfer of a coracoid graft and conjoined tendon over the top of the lower subscapularis tendon results in increased tension in the inferior fibers of the subscapularis, enhancing anterior stability;
- sling effect: conjoined tendon forms a sling across the anterior-inferior capsule when the shoulder is in 90° abduction and 90° external rotation, providing additional soft tissue restraint anteriorly, all of which act to prevent engagement of the Hill-Sachs lesion even before the anterior capsule is repaired;
- capsular effect: follows capsular restoration.

Shoulder instability is one of most controversial joint diseases in terms of diagnosis and treatment. Several open surgical treatments for primary anterior glenohumeral instability have been published, including long-term follow-up of these methods, which are reliable and time-tested and can yield excellent clinical results [3]. The use of arthroscopy has improved the recognition of pathologic findings in shoulder instability and allowed a better understanding of the anatomopathology of instability and the correlation between symptoms and lesions. The arthroscopic technique allows reparative and reconstructive surgical procedures aimed at selective treatment of the injured structures, obviating tenotomy or splitting of the subscapularis, thus reducing the risk of iatrogenic damage. In international literature, some studies demonstrate the results of arthroscopic treatment of recurrent traumatic anterior instability comparable with those achieved historically with open procedures [4].

Despite these exciting advances, open surgery remains an acceptable method of treatment, particularly when a surgeon lacks the equipment, experience, or technical skills needed to perform an arthroscopic repair. Moreover, open surgery remains the preferred method of treatment in situations in which arthroscopic techniques cannot adequately address the anatomic lesion, such as anterior instability in the presence of glenoid and/or humeral bony defects or soft tissue deficiencies.

There are two basic types of surgical treatment for shoulders with anterior instability: anatomic and nonanatomic. The goals of the anatomic repairs (open or arthroscopic) are to restore the labrum to its normal position and to obtain the appropriate tension in the capsule-ligaments complex [5]. The goal of nonanatomic surgical procedures is to stabilize the shoulder by compensating for the capsule-labral and osseous injury with an osseous graft that blocks excessive translation and restores stability [1, 6]. Several studies [7] have demonstrated excellent outcomes with nonanatomic stabilizations, but there are reports that show complications, such as loss of motion, recurrent instability, and arthritis [8–10]. These nonanatomic procedures are mostly used by European surgeons, whereas many North American surgeons avoid them as a first approach [11, 12]. This is a crucial point between European and American techniques, as the the latter use nonanatomic procedures in the presence of a bony defect >20–23% on the glenoid side. European surgeons generally adopt the principles of the French school, in which procedures such as the Latarjet are used not only in the presence of bone loss (both glenoid and humeral side, i.e., glenoid track), but also when capsular deficiency is present or after several dislocations, when soft tissue mechanical properties may change and become more pronounced. The negative aspect of these types of procedures is related to the new anatomy. In these cases, revision surgery can be challenging; however, when these procedures are performed appropriately by well-trained surgeons, good results can generally be obtained.

3.2 Patient Selection

Preoperative evaluation of the patient is the crucial point by which to determine the best method of treatment. Based upon history, clinical examination, imaging evaluation, and patient demand, it is possible to find elements to determine whether the patient should be submitted to rehabilitation, arthroscopy, or open-shoulder stabilization. Important information is cause, number, and frequency of episodes; direction of instability; force of trauma; and arm position at the time of initial injury. Mechanical symptoms, such as catching or locking, may suggest a displaced labral tear or osseous defect. Instability that occurs in the midrange of motion or during sleep suggests an osseous defect that overcomes muscular restraint. Neuromuscular assessment should be performed because axillary nerve injury could occur during traumatic anterior instability.

Studies have shown that physical examination for anterior shoulder instability is clinically helpful if the criterion for a positive test is the reproduction of a symptom of instability [13]. A positive sulcus sign in external rotation is suggestive of multidirectional instability, and closure of rotator interval is suggested [14–16]. Apprehension sign relieved by a relocation maneuver (relocation test) can be diagnostic of anteroinferior shoulder instability [17]. With the load-and-shift test, it is possible to assess the grade and direction of shoulder laxity/instability [16, 18]. Asymptomatic laxity in any direction if used as a criterion for instability can substantially change the number of patients given that diagnosis [13].

3.3 Imaging

Our series of X-rays is based on true anteroposterior (AP) (in neutral, internal, and external rotation) and axillary views that help detect relevant glenoid fractures, Hill-Sachs lesions, or associated fractures [19]. Magnetic resonance (MR) can confirm the presence of a Bankart lesion. ArthroMR can help determine the presence of an associated superior labral anterior-posterior (SLAP) lesion but can be useful when rare but important lesions, such as humeral avulsions of the glenohumeral ligaments (HAGL lesion) or capsular ruptures are present. This information is important for the technical difficulty involved in arthroscopic repair of these types of injuries and because the correct surgery planning may reduce the rate of recurrence in these cases if lesions are addressed by arthroscopy.

In patients >40 years with shoulder instability, rotator cuff tear should be suspected, especially after an anteroinferior or inferior dislocation. Computed tomography (CT) with 3D reconstructions can be helpful when bone deficiency is suspected. This type of study best demonstrates the presence of an acute or chronic condition, amount of bone loss, and extent of the lesion [20].

3.4 Surgery

When surgery is recommended, most cases of anterior-inferior glenohumeral instability can be treated with either open or arthroscopic approaches because there is substantial overlap in the indications for these procedures, except in the presence of engaging bone-loss lesions [2]. In patients with multidirectional instability, which requires both anterior and posterior capsular shift, the first option to consider is arthroscopy. However, despite advances in shoulder arthroscopy, there are still several relative contraindications to the procedure. These include bone loss, humeral avulsions of the glenohumeral ligaments (HAGL), and capsular lesions. Other relative indications for open surgery include a previously failed arthroscopic or open repair. The essential lesion in a shoulder with traumatic anterior instability is a Bankart lesion, which usually occurs with some degree of capsular injury or stretch [21]. Primary dislocation in young, active people, can be repaired arthroscopically when neither capsular deficiency nor large bone loss are present.

The appropriate treatment of anterior-inferior instability in young patients participating in contact sports remains controversial. In such cases with engaging bone-loss lesions, we prefer the Latarjet procedure [22], for which excellent results have been reported [23–25]. From a general point of view, we follow the Instability Severity Index Score (ISIS) described by Balg and Boileau [26] to better determine which patients are appropriate for open or arthroscopic procedure. The score (0–10) is based on a preoperative questionnaire, clinical examination, and radiographs to identify significant or pertinent risk factors and includes six significant preoperative factors:

- age at time of surgery (<20 years);
- preoperative degree of sport participation;
- preoperative type of sport;
- presence of shoulder hyperlaxity;
- Hill-Sachs lesion present on an anteroposterior radiograph with the shoulder in external rotation;
- loss of sclerotic inferior glenoid contour in AP view.

The categories "patient <20 years" and "involved in competitive sports" score two points each; "contact or forced overhead activities" scores one point; "anterior or inferior hyperlaxity" scores one point. On AP radiograph, two points are added if a Hill-Sachs lesion is visible on external rotation and two points if there is loss of the normal inferior glenoid contour. If the ISIS score is more than six points, the risk of recurrence after arthroscopic Bankart repair is 70%. Consequently, an open procedure such as the Latarjet procedure [1] is the best option. Careful discussion with the patient is of paramount importance to determine his or her desires regarding quality of future sport activity and acceptable rate of recurrence.

3.4.1 Exposure Technique

We use the deltopectoral approach. A 5-cm skin incision is made starting at the tip of the coracoid process and extending inferiorly. Placing a self-retaining retractor between the pectoralis major and the deltoid and a Hohmann-type retractor over the top of the coracoid process aids in surgical exposure (Fig. 3.1a).

Tips and Tricks

During tenotomy of the pectoralis minor muscle, and especially during resection of the coracoacromial ligament, attention must be paid to protecting the subscapularis tendon situated immediately under the apophysis, inserting a surgical instrument (Fig. 3.1b) as protection under the coracoacromial ligament. Another important procedure is accurately freeing the base of the coracoid, which must be uncovered as far as its curvature, in order to perform an osteotomy sufficient for obtaining a bone block about 2-cm long. Care must also be taken in freeing the clavipectoral fascia from the conjoined tendon, which will remain inserted at the top of the coracoid graft itself. Indeed, in the region medial to the conjoined tendon are the coracoid vessels and nerves and the musculocutaneous nerve, and it is important to protect them from any iatrogenic damage. A special Hohmann-type retractor will aid in obtaining the best possible exposure of the coracoid. It is important to use flat-ended Hohmann-type retractors with short spikes that can grasp the bone to expose it properly in the limited space offered by the surgical access. A special autostatic retractor is useful in such cases.

Complications

- Insufficient exposure of the coracoid, which may have a negative effect on the osteotomy;
- damage of the subscapularis tendon during coracoacromial ligament resection;
- iatrogenic damage to nerves and vessels at the level of the medial part of the coracoid.

Fig. 3.1a, b. Anterior view of the left shoulder. Coracoid position after a modified deltopectoral approach. **a** A retractor is placed on the base of the bone. **b** The coracoid process is freed from coracoacromial ligament laterally and from pectoralis minor tendon medially

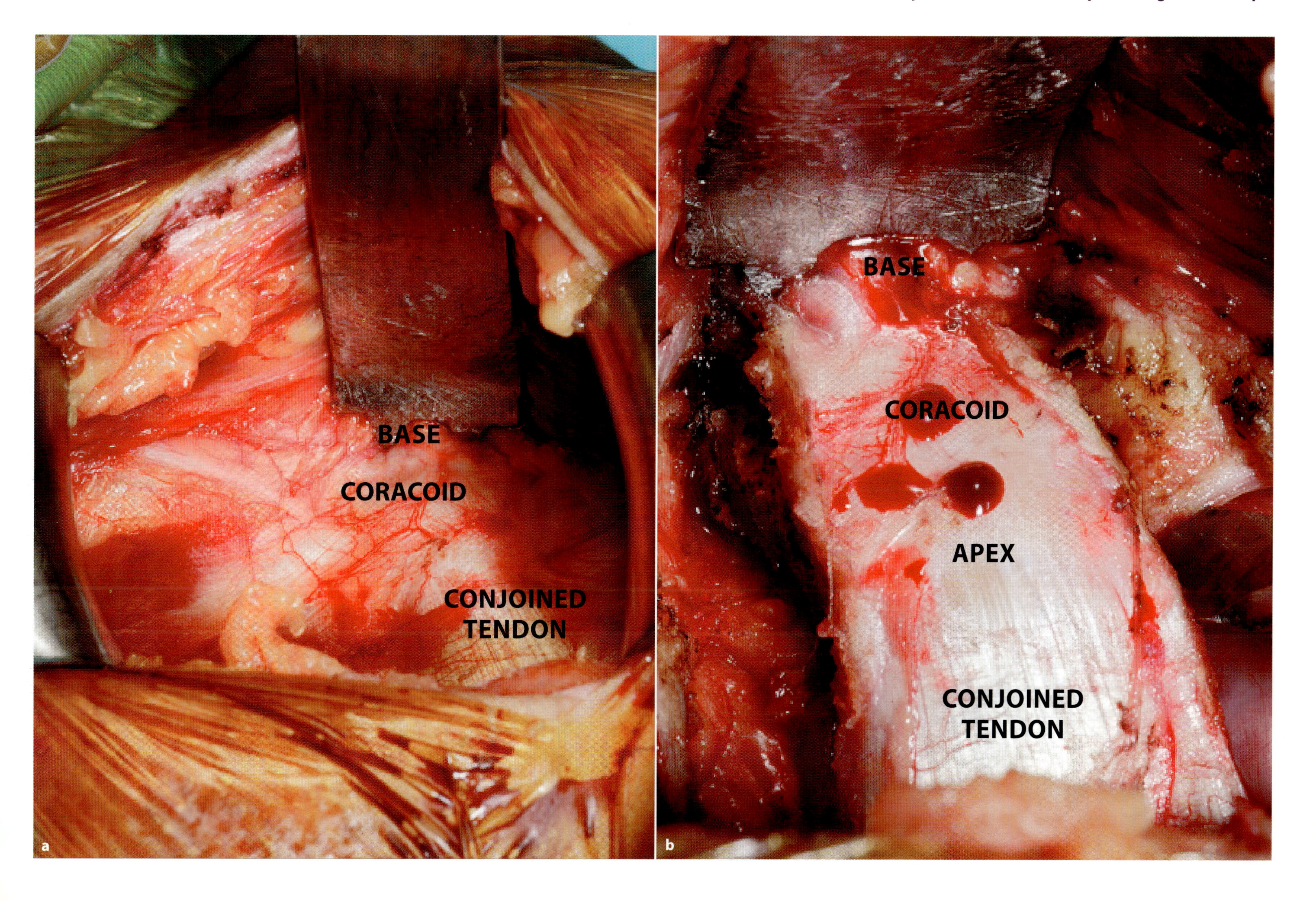
BASE
CORACOID
CONJOINED
TENDON
a
BASE
CORACOID
APEX
CONJOINED
TENDON
b

3.4.2 Coracoid Osteotomy

The coracoacromial ligament is released from the lateral side of the coracoid process, and the pectoralis minor tendon attachment is released on its medial side. Care must be taken with the subscapularis muscle of the coracoid process underneath. Osteotomy of the coracoid process at the level of the "knee" is performed with a microsagittal 90°-angled blade saw (Fig. 3.2). The conjoined tendon is left attached to the coracoid graft.

Tips and Tricks

It is useful to keep the sagittal saw cool with saline solution to reduce the temperature created during cutting. It is important to remember that the osteotomy plane of the coracoid crosses the proximal region of the glenoid, so it is advisable to avoid moving medially during the osteotomy because this could harm the glenoid itself and the soft tissues in the proximal region of the joint. It is useful to direct the reciprocating saw from the medial region to the lateral region of the coracoid, or, if this is difficult because of limited space, keep it vertical. It is important to use short blades of approximately 2-cm wide. A 2-cm-diameter scalpel may be useful for terminating the osteotomy of the coracoid in the deepest region to avoid losing control of the last phases of the cutting procedure.

Complications

- Damage to the glenoid in the proximal region due to an incorrect osteotomy;
- possible damage to the vascular/nerve structures of the medial region of the coracoid;
- overheating of the bone in the osteotomy region, with damage to blood vessels (possible integration problems due to insufficient vascular flow).

Fig. 3.2. Osteotomy of the coracoid process at the level of the "knee" with a microsagittal 90°-angled blade saw. A Hohmann-type retractor on the base of the coracoid process helps to cut the bone very close to the "knee" to create a large graft

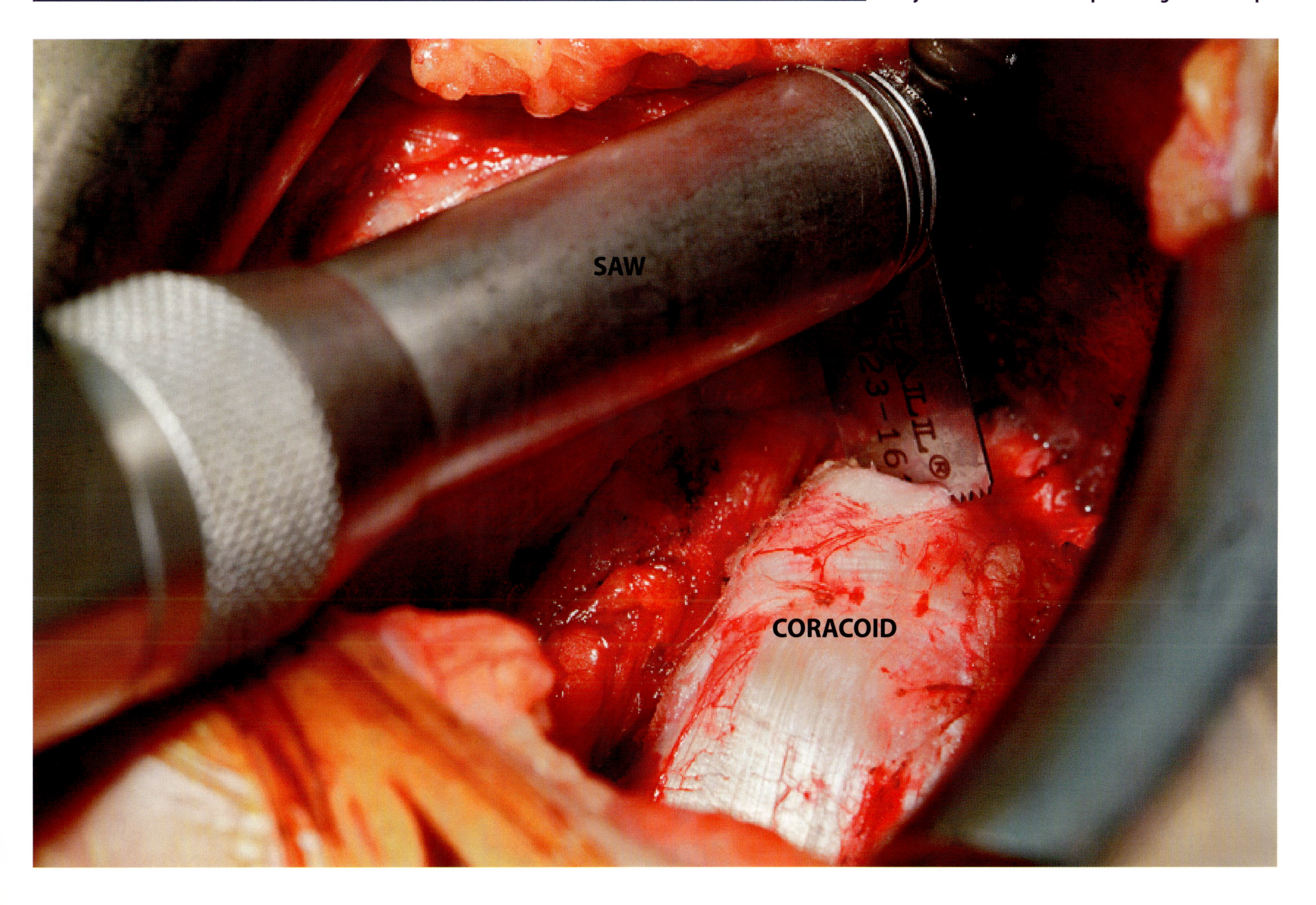
SAW
CORACOID

3.4.3 Coracoid Preparation

As shown in Figure 3.3a, the coracoid graft is well exposed and has been carefully freed from soft tissues. The conjoined tendon, totally intact, is inserted at the top of the bone block. Proper coracoid exposure will help when preparing the holes for correct insertion of the screws for bone fixation. It can be useful to free the surface of the dorsal region (Fig. 3.3b) of the coracoid from the periosteum to expose it properly, but for biological and vascularization reasons, it is advisable to keep it in place and bore the holes through the soft tissue. We use the bone block without making any rotations. Its deep region is placed at the level of the inferior part of the glenoid neck to obtain the best bone-to-bone match for optimal healing.

Tips and Tricks

To obtain good exposure of the dorsal region of the coracoid and show the bony surface of the graft, it can be useful to remove the periosteum and soft tissues (Fig. 3.3b). The dorsal region of the graft often has a very particular conformation and often differs from patient to patient. Using dedicated forceps that grasp securely (Fig. 3.3a, b) for gripping the bone block can aid movement without the risk of tearing and twisting.

Complications

- Anomalous stretching of the conjoined tendon, with stretching of nerves and vessels in the tendon region;
- damage to the conjoined tendon.

Fig. 3.3a, b. **a** Coracoid bone graft is completely freed from soft tissue. **b** Cleaning the dorsal surface of the bone it is important to prepare for the next steps of the procedure

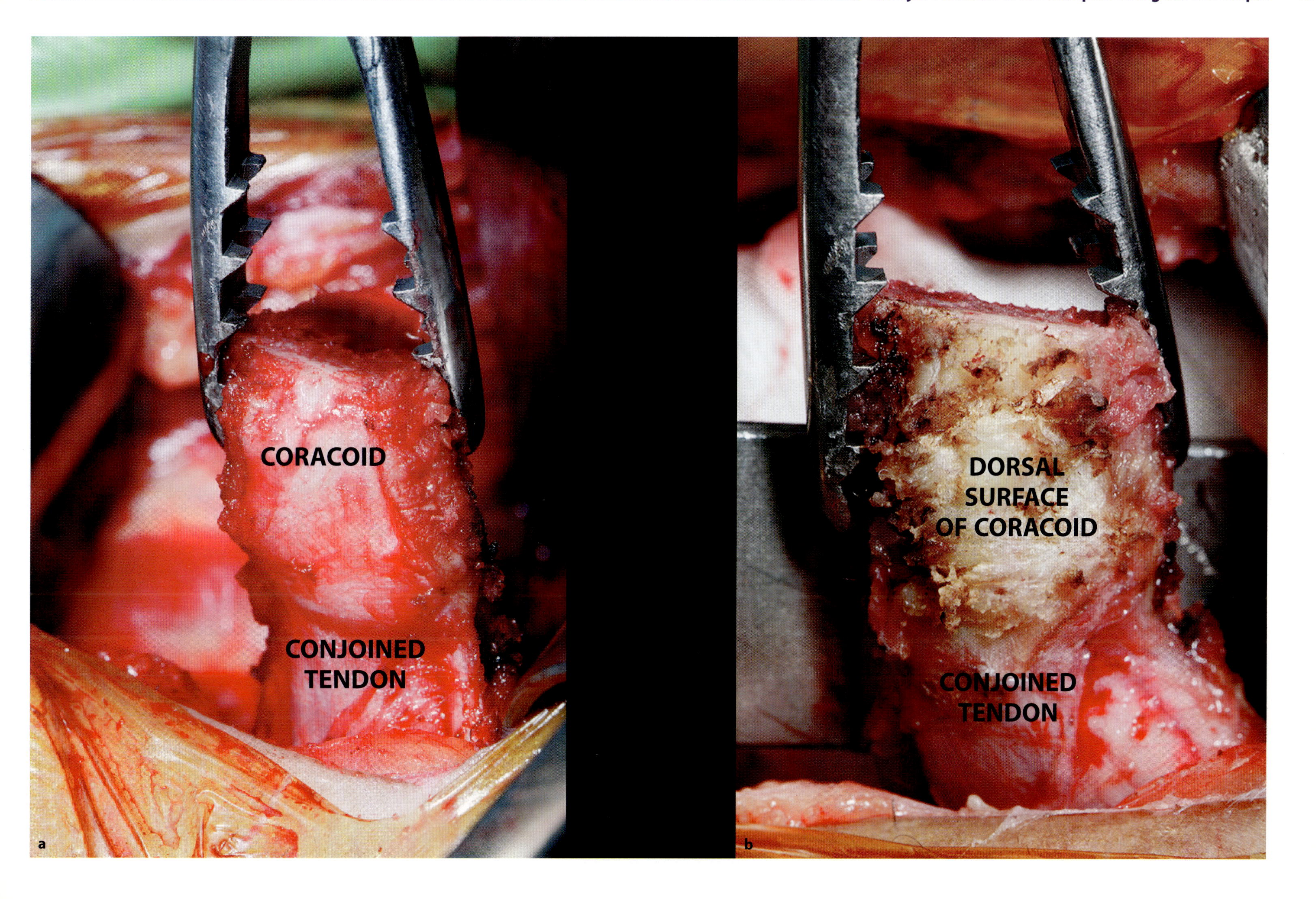
CORACOID
CONJOINED TENDON
a
DORSAL SURFACE OF CORACOID
CONJOINED TENDON
b

3.4.4 Coracoid Preparation

The microsagittal saw and high-speed burr are then used to decorticate the deep surface of the coracoid bone graft (Fig. 3.4a). Here again, sterile saline solution is useful to reduce the heat caused by the saw during cutting. Exposing the cancellous bone will indicate that decortication has been performed correctly. Bleeding from cancellous bone will improve integration of the bone graft on the glenoid neck (Fig. 3.4b).

Tips and Tricks

It is important not to remove a great deal of bony tissue during the osteotomy and above all not to make dangerous maneuvers in the most distal region, where the conjoined tendon is attached (Fig. 3.4b).

Complications

- Removing too much cortical bone may weaken the bone graft, which could break during subsequent bone fixation;
- overheating caused by the reciprocating saw while cutting could reduce or interrupt the local microbleeding that is useful for bone integration;
- possible damage to the attachment of the conjoined tendon at the moment of decortication of the deep surface of the coracoid.

Fig. 3.4a, b. **a** Preparation of the deep surface of the coracoid process. **b** The cancellus bone is exposed with a straight saw to obtain bone bleeding and flattening

a
SAW
b
CORACOID
DEEP SURFACE

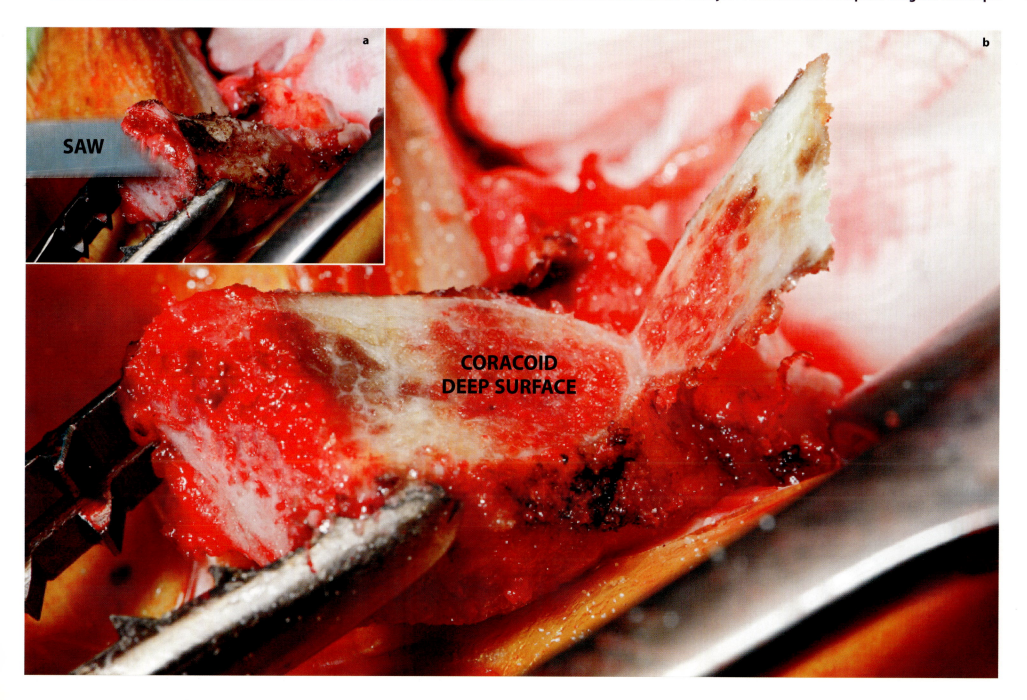

3.4.5 Coracoid Preparation

The drill guide, via the guide wire (Fig. 3.5), allows the surgeon to create two dorsal-ventral holes in the coracoid graft using the 3.5-mm drill perpendicular to its long axis. The coracoid graft is then placed and kept under the pectoralis major muscle during the rest of the procedure. Figure 3.5 shows the specific pointer for the metal wires used as a guide, which will permit inserting the two screws at an exact distance apart in the subsequent bone-fixation phase. The guide has a distance between centers equal to that of the wedged profile plate that will be used later. The parallel positioning of the two wires guarantees that the two screws are positioned perfectly parallel.

Tips and Tricks

To obtain correct exposure of the dorsal surface of the coracoid, it is useful to remove a small amount of the dorsal periosteum. Dedicated forceps with a secure grip is the solution for holding the graft perfectly stable to drill the holes. Avoiding stretching the conjoined tendon will prevent damage to the musculocutaneous nerve that passes through the tendon a few centimeters (approximately 5.5 cm) distally from the coracoid attachment [27, 28].

Complications

- Incorrect positioning of the coracoid holes could create difficulties implanting the screws and the wedged profile plate;
- nonparallel insertion of the wires could cause the drilling of nonparallel holes and thus incorrect positioning of the screws during bone fixation;
- too much traction on the conjoined tendon could case apraxia of the musculocutaneous nerve.

Fig. 3.5. With a special guide by Arthrex, the two Kirschner wires are inserted parallel from dorsal to deep surface of the bone graft to prepare parallel holes for inserting the screws at the end of the procedure

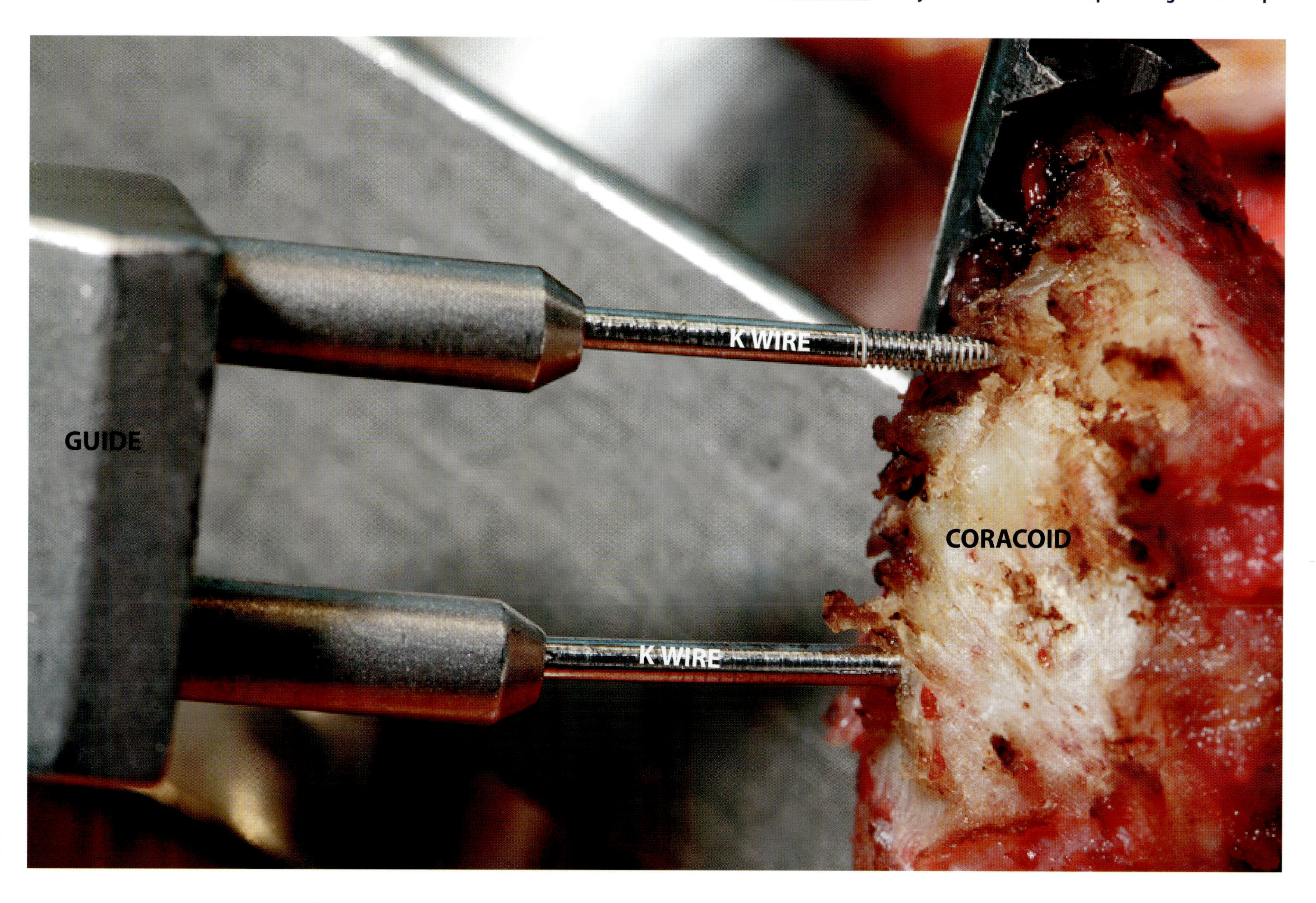
K WIRE
GUIDE
CORACOID
K WIRE

3.4.6 Splitting the Subscapularis Tendon

With the shoulder in external rotation, the subscapularis muscle is divided in line with its fibers at the junction of the fibers between the upper two thirds and lower one third of the muscle using electrocautery, being careful to avoid damage to the biceps tendon laterally and joint capsule underneath. To improve capsular exposure, using a Gelpi retractor is helpful (Fig. 3.6) [23, 24]. If the patient exhibits a major constitutional laxity, the subscapularis will be divided at the junction between the upper half and lower half of the muscle in order to obtain greater stability due to the action of the muscle mass itself [23, 24].

Tips and Tricks

It is advisable to use a dressing with a Vicryl drawstring, which, if placed between the scapular body and the subscapularis muscle, will help reduce bleeding and improve visualization of the glenoid neck. Absolute respect for fibers of the subscapularis muscle during the split will help with early shoulder rehabilitation. Not extending the split too far medially will prevent damage to nerve structures (subscapularis nerve).

Complications

- Damage to the pulley and long head of the biceps tendon with lateral extension of subscapularis tendon split;
- damage to one of the subscapularis nerve branches with medial extension of the subscapularis fibers split.

Fig. 3.6. Anterior view of left shoulder. The subscapularis muscle is split with a Gelpi retractor, and the capsule is exposed

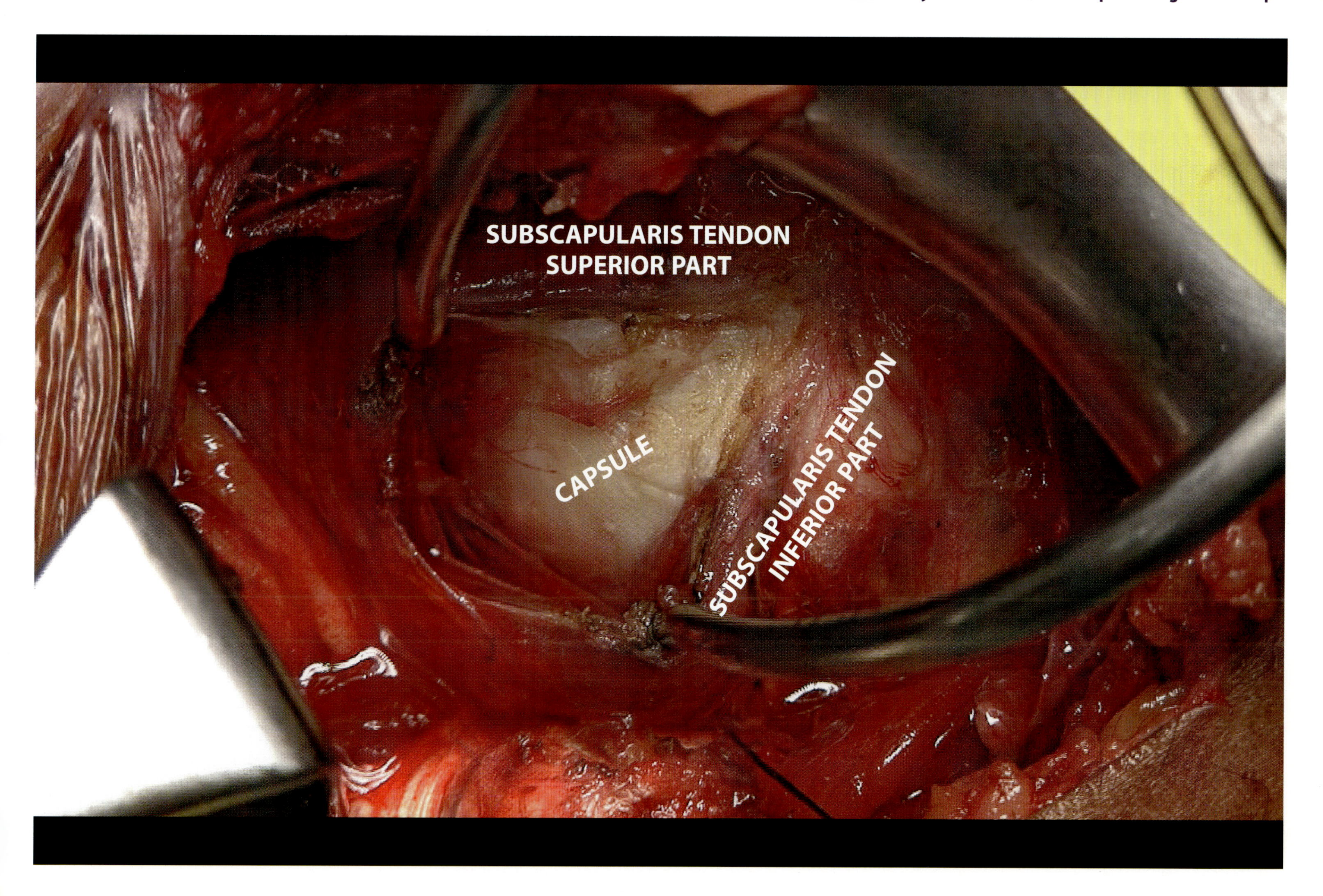
SUBSCAPULARIS TENDON
SUPERIOR PART
CAPSULE
SUBSCAPULARIS TENDON
INFERIOR PART

3.4.7 Capsulotomy

A horizontal (east-west) capsulotomy is performed parallel to the incision of the subscapularis to expose the shoulder joint (Fig. 3.7). In the medial region, exactly at the attachment of the capsule on the labrum, the capsule is carefully detached in the cranial/caudal fashion, thus exposing the glenoid region, where the coracoid bone graft will be implanted. At this point, two retractors are used: a standard Fukuda retractor laterally for the humeral head, and a forked glenoid-type retractor placed on the anterior scapular neck as medially as possible to improve visualization of the site of graft insertion.

Tips and Tricks

The capsulotomy must reflect the opening of the subscapularis fibers. An east-west capsulotomy is also useful for the possible optional repair of the capsule itself at the end of the surgery. Accurate detachment from the glenoid will preserve the most important part of the capsule for possible repair. For capsule incision, it is recommended that a long-handled scalpel (no. 11) be used, obtaining a moderate posterior subluxation of the humeral head with the aid of an assistant. After accessing the glenoid labrum and performing disinsertion at the glenoid, it is useful to insert a Fukuda retractor into the joint to pull the humeral head laterally, moving the arm in internal rotation, and a forked Hohmann-type retractor into the medial region of the glenoid neck. It is useful to remove all other retractors to obtain optimal visualization of the glenoid neck, which is the key point in this step of the procedure.

Complications

- A capsulotomy performed without good visualization could lead to damage to the underlying cartilage;
- partial or insufficient capsulotomy could prevent insertion of the described retractors, which optimize the view of the surgical field.

Fig. 3.7. The capsule is opened in the same direction as the subscapularis split. It is important to avoid lateral damage of the long head of biceps pulley. Clear exposition of the joint can avoid damage to the humeral-head cartilage and glenoid

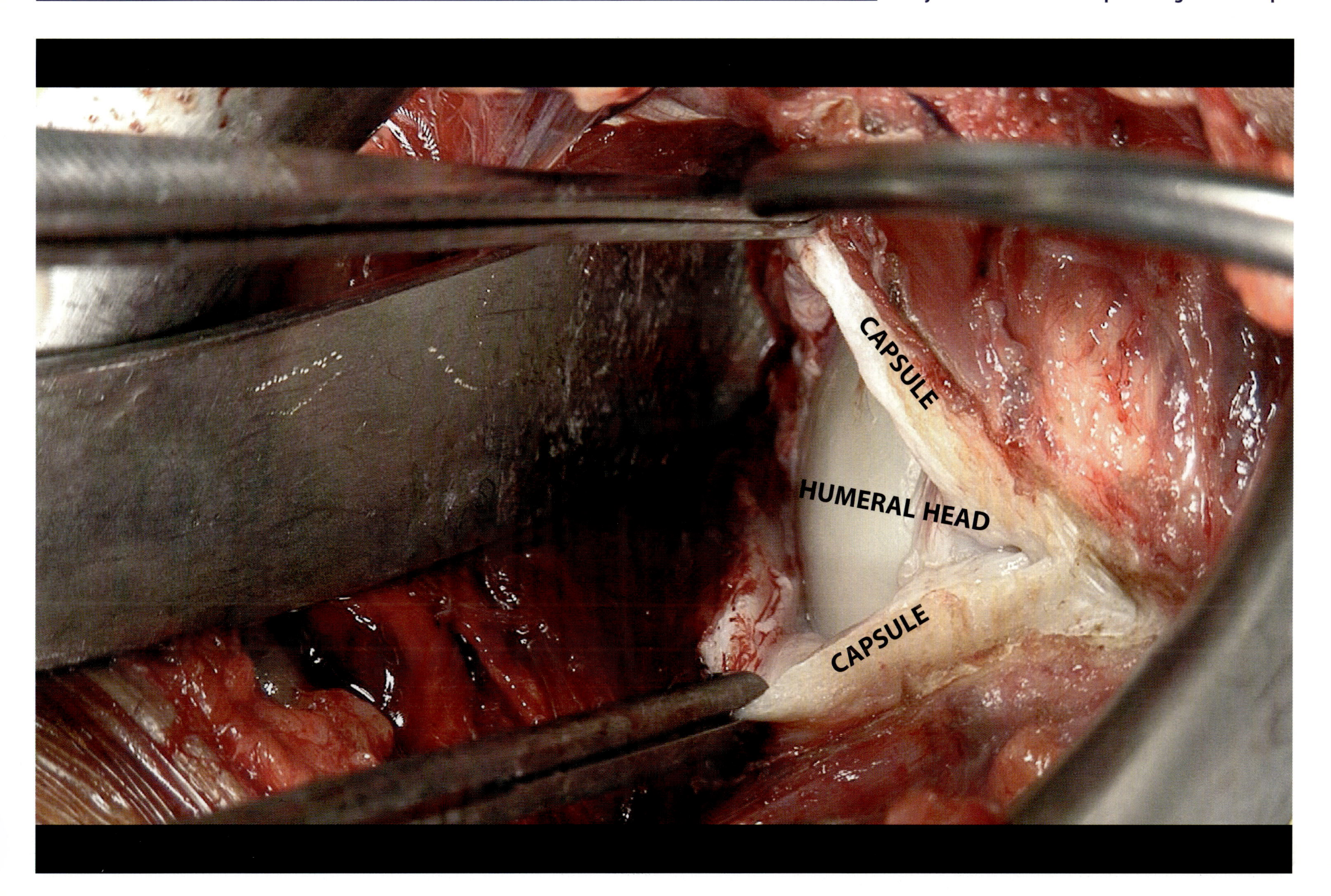
CAPSULE
HUMERAL HEAD
CAPSULE

3.4.8 Glenoid Preparation

The anteroinferior glenoid rim surface is cleared of soft tissue Fig. 3.8a). With a high-speed burr, the anteroinferior glenoid neck is prepared for placement of the coracoid bone graft (Fig. 3.8b). The good exposure of the glenoid obtained with the use of the specific retractors, described above, makes it possible to obtain the best view of the surgical field. To handle the upper portion of the subscapularis muscle, we use a swan retractor devised by Atrhrex. The anterior-inferior region of the glenoid neck is prepared to obtain bleeding from the bone and to attain correct leveling of the surface to aid the bone-to-bone contact between glenoid and coracoid graft.

Tips and Tricks

The choice of retractors is important. In this phase, only a humeral-head retractor (Fukuda) is used in the lateral region, a forked glenoid-type retractor medially, and a swan retractor devised by Arthrex for the upper portion of the subscapularis. The upper limb is positioned in neutral rotation.

Complications

- Poor decortication of the anteroinferior surface of the glenoid neck, with little bleeding, could reduce the possibility of integration of the coracoid bone graft;
- incorrect flattering of the glenoid bone surface could reduce the contact between the glenoid and coracoid graft and jeopardize bone integration.

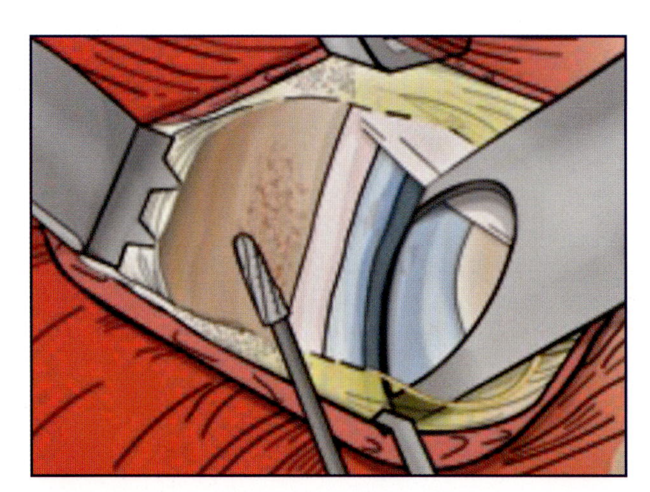

Glenoid neck preparation with high speed burr

Fig. 3.8a, b. Glenoid preparation: **a** the anteroinferior glenoid neck is cleared of the soft tissue, and **b** with a high-speed burr, bleeding from the bone is created

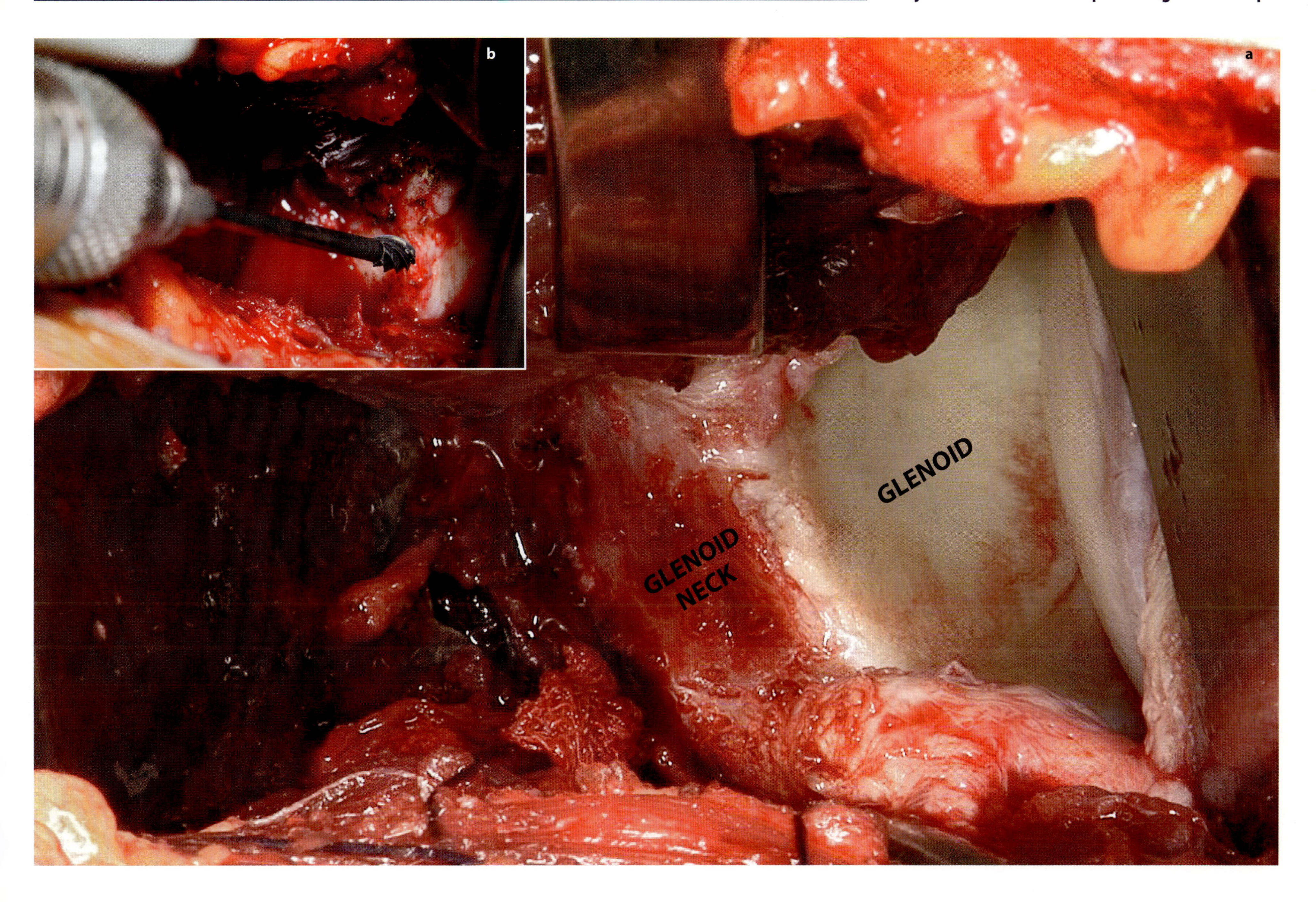
b
a
GLENOID
GLENOID
NECK

3.4.9 Glenoid Preparation

The first guide wire is inserted for subsequent drilling of the holes through the glenoid. The first wire to be inserted is the lower one (Fig. 3.9) in order to obtain correct positioning of the lower screw and therefore of the entire implant. In fact, positioning of the second guide (superior) wire, screws, and coracoid implant in the final phase all depend on placement of the first wire. For this reason, it must be performed with absolute precision.

Tips and Tricks

A 0.9-mm K-wire with threaded apical region is used, supplied by the manufacturer of the screws. It is important to position the first guide wire while precisely observing the lower glenoid margin to ensure that the distal screw will not be implanted too far down. The coracoid graft offset (Fig. 3.9) will be established, attempting, after implantation of the K-wire, to insert the specific guide on the implanted wire. Generally speaking, the coracoid has a lateromedial surface of approximately 2 cm. Therefore, the first wire will be implanted approximately 1 cm medially from the lateral edge of the glenoid. The guide wire must be positioned parallel to the joint surface of the glenoid to avoid positioning the screws inside the joint in the following phase, which would cause serious damage to cartilage surfaces.

Complications

- Lateral or medial implantation of the guide wire;
- implantation of the first guide wire too low or too high;
- implantation of the first guide wire not parallel to the glenoid joint surface.

Fig. 3.9. The first Kirschner wire (*inferior*) is placed. The offset is established, evaluating the width of the coracoid graft

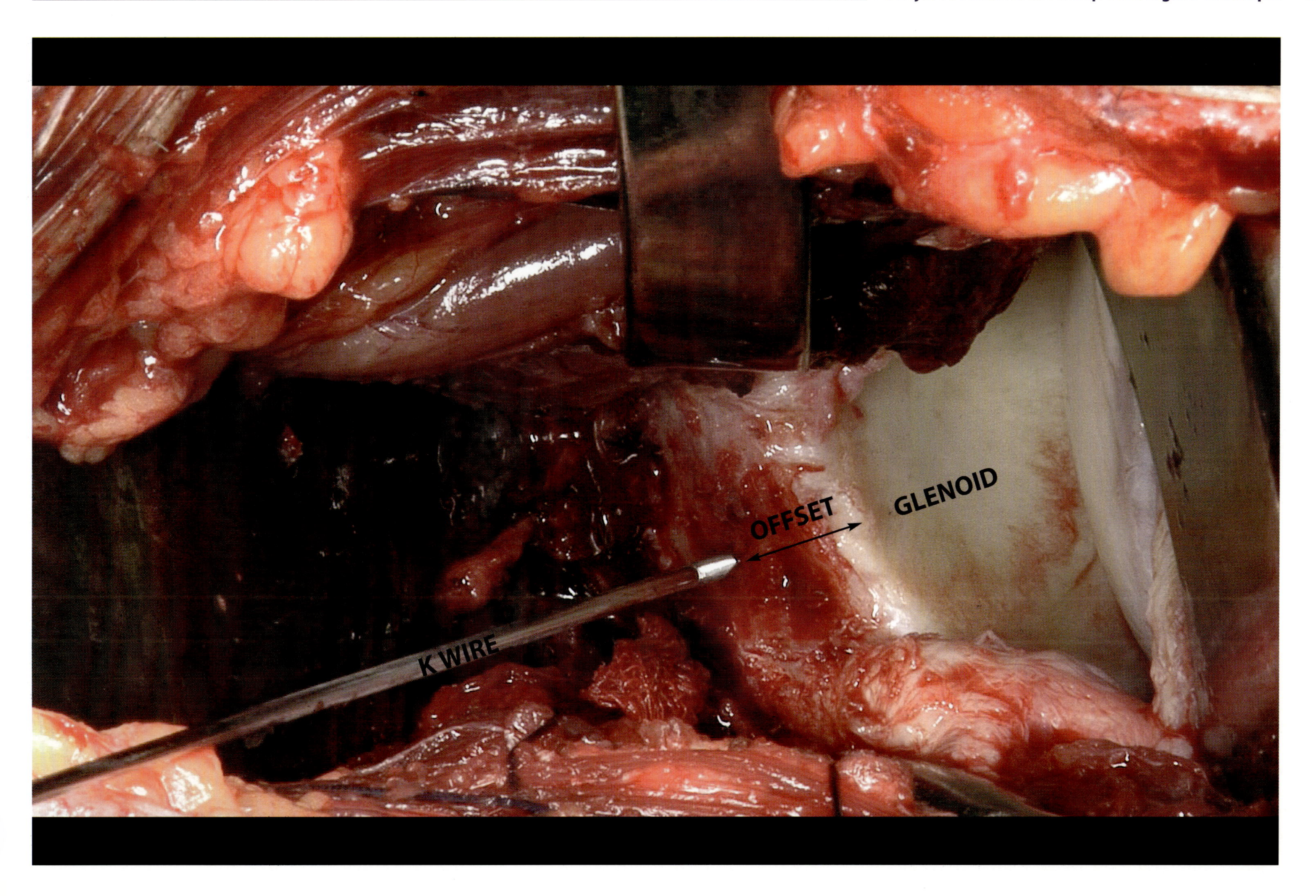
GLENOID
OFFSET
K WIRE

3.4.10 Glenoid Preparation

The second 0.9-mm K-wire with its guide (Fig. 3.10b) is positioned, with indication of the offset if used. The first wire inserted will determine the position for the second wire (Fig. 3.10a). The guide is useful for positioning the two wires at the correct distance between centers so as to insert the two screws and the wedged profile plate.

Tips and Tricks

The guide is useful for evaluating the offset in this phase, before drilling the transglenoid holes (Fig. 3.10c). Both wires must be positioned parallel in order to avoid later malpositioning of the bone graft.

Complications

- Implantation not parallel to the glenoid joint surface of the guide wires can interfere with screw positioning, leading to joint protrusion and shear stress force on the coracoid graft;
- implantation of the second K-wire too laterally (poor offset), with the bone graft protruding beyond the joint space in the final phase.

Fig. 3.10a-c. a The second Kirschner wire is placed with the help of the **b** special guide from Arthrex. **c** The drill is used to create the two holes on the glenoid neck

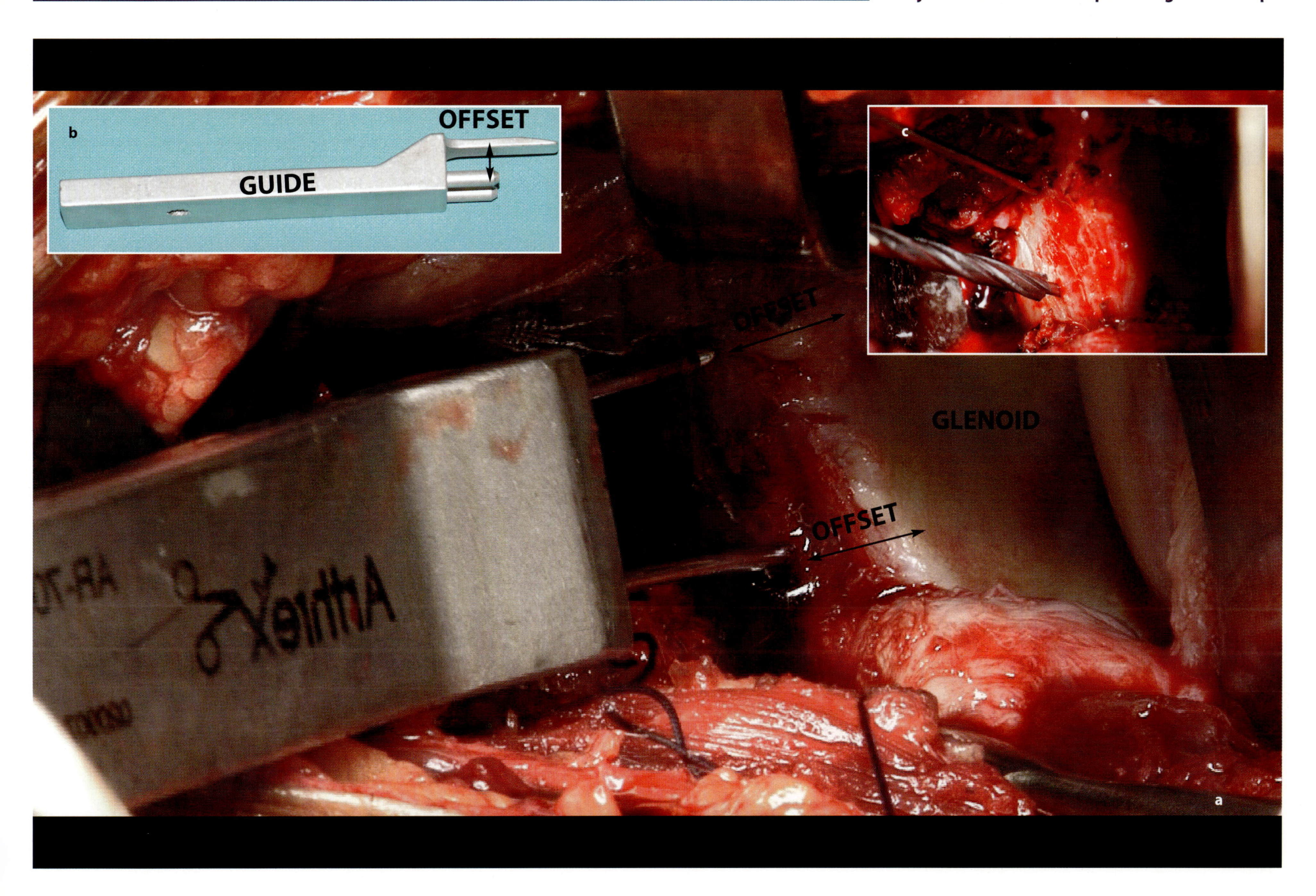
b
OFFSET
GUIDE
c
OFFSET
GLENOID
OFFSET
Arthrex
a

3.4.11 Miniplate (Wedged Profile Plate)

To obtain better compression and load distribution between the coracoid graft and glenoid bone surface, we designed a miniplate (wedged profile plate; Arthrex Inc, Naples, FL, USA) (Fig. 3.11a), the characteristics of which each correspond to a specific biomechanical function appropriate for the Latarjet procedure. The figure-of-eight configuration allows for better torsional orientation of the plate on the dorsal coracoid bone-graft surface. This allows the plate to distribute the load evenly throughout the bone, avoiding stress risers that occur when screws only are used. When compressed during the screwing phase, the miniplate, positioned with the wedge profile oriented medially (Fig. 3.11b), will tilt the coracoid bone graft in that direction, aligning the bone contact surface between the coracoid graft and the steep glenoid neck. Four spikes on the plate are designed to hold the graft as a whole and to reduce traction forces from the conjoined tendon, at the same time improving plate and graft stability during surgical fixation: plate-coracoid-glenoid neck. The more the bone loss, the less steep is the glenoid neck. In this situation, the improved compression force effect from the plate is more important than the wedge effect. The wedge is useful in minor bone loss because of the steeper glenoid neck.

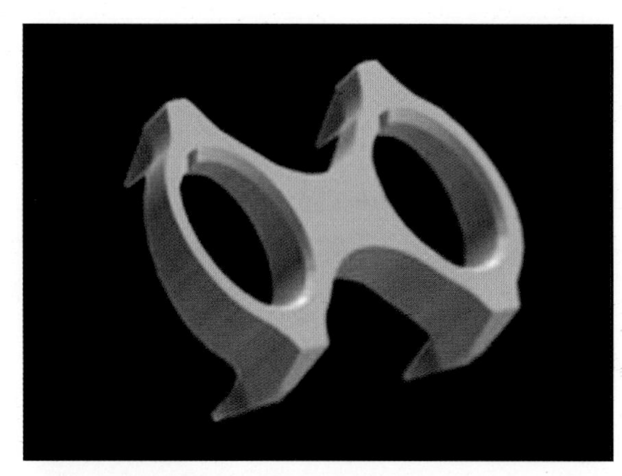

Wedged Profile Plate (Arthrex Inc, Naples, FL)

Fig. 3.11a, b. a The wedged profile plate is placed on the coracoid graft. **b** The wedged profile is placed in medial part of the graft

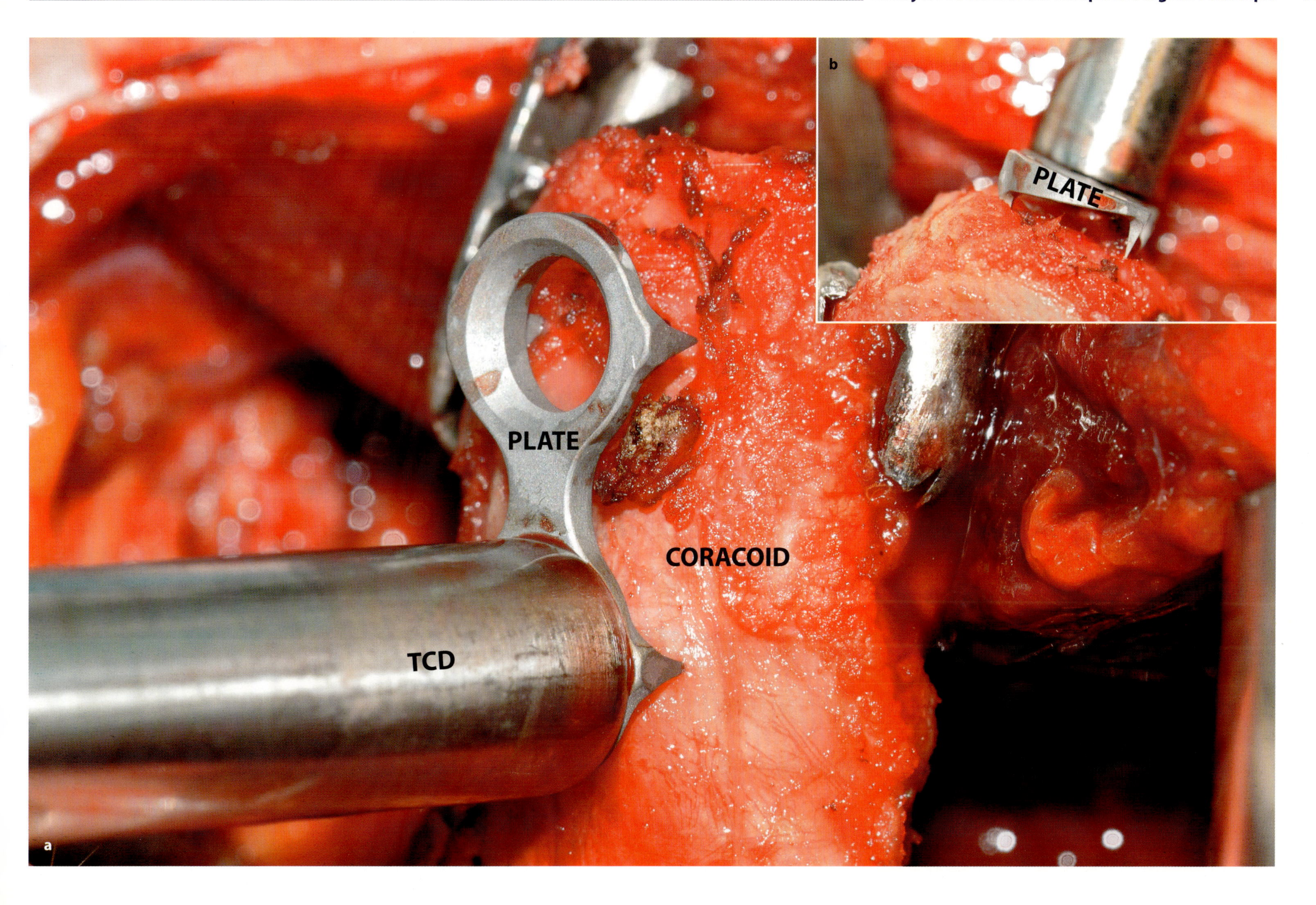
b
PLATE
PLATE
CORACOID
TCD
a

3.4.11.1 Plate Technique

The coracoid graft is retrieved from under the pectoralis major and held with grasping forceps. The wedged profile plate, with its thickest margin placed medially, is centered with respect to the coracoid graft width and height and stabilized by the presence of the spikes on the plate. In this phase, it is advisable to be certain that the plate holes are centered over the bone graft holes to avoid a shift in the bone graft position when it is being screwed into place.

Tips and Tricks

A cannulated temporary compression device (TCD) is used to stabilize the plate over the coracoid graft through the lower drilled hole (Fig. 3.12b-d). The TCD is used like a joystick. Positioning a guide wire in the upper bone hole helps keep the plate in place on the bone graft while the TCD is being screwed onto the coracoid graft (Fig. 3.12d).

Complications

- Incorrect positioning of the wedge of the plate;
- pulling with the grasper punch or with the TCD positioning the graft too far cranially could damage the musculocutaneous nerve that crosses through the short head of the biceps and coracobrachialis muscles.

Fig. 3.12a-d. The cannulated temporary compression device is placed to stabilize the plate and guide the graft against the glenoid neck, like a joystick, with the two Kirschner wires. Image sequence clarifies the exact method of placing the coracoid graft on the glenoid neck

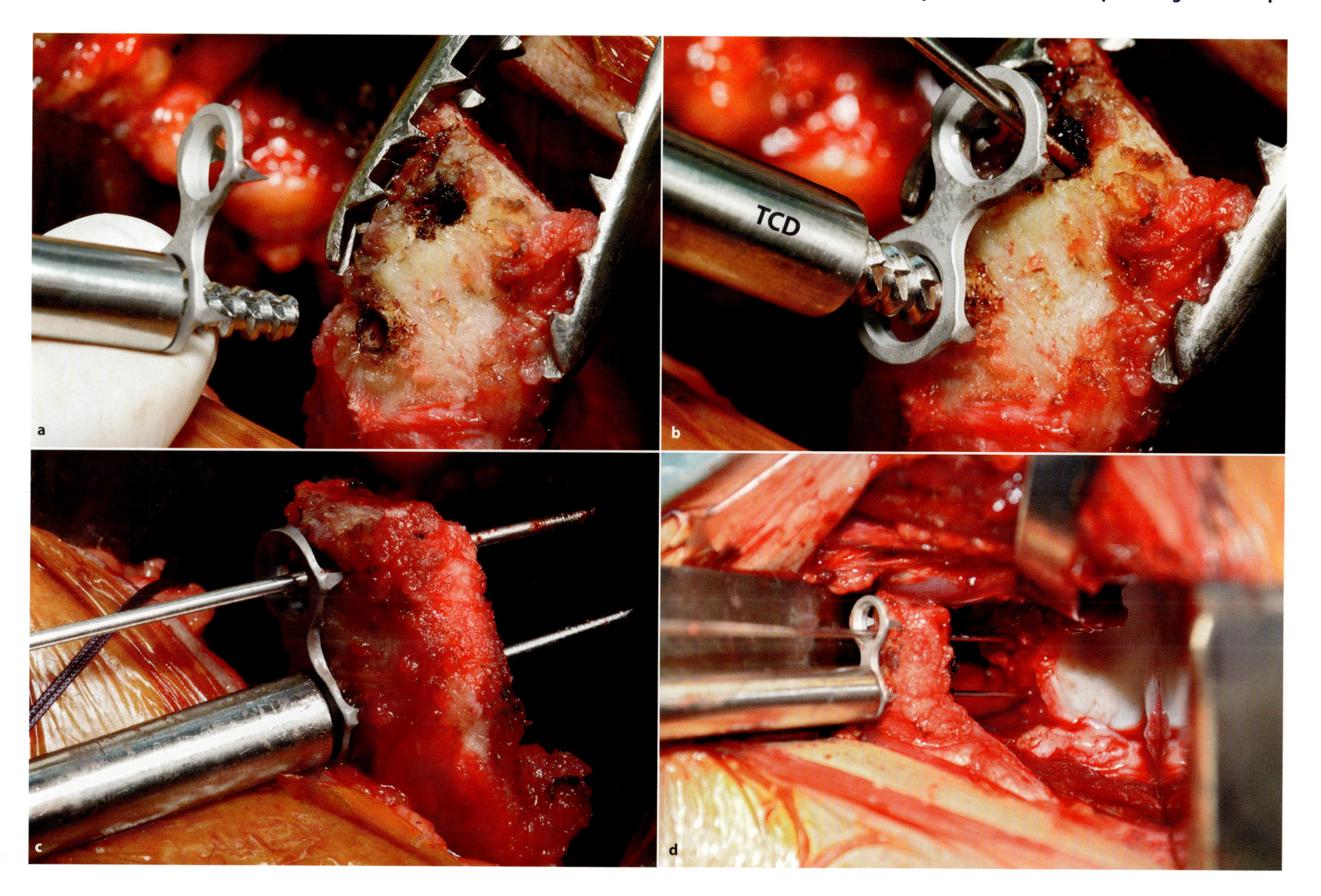
a
b
TCD
c
d

3.4.11.2 Plate Technique

A partially threaded 3.75-mm screw (length usually between 34 and 38 mm) is inserted first through the upper coracoid screw hole (Fig. 3.13a, b). The TCD is then removed, leaving the K-wire as a guide for a 3.75-mm cannulated screw through the lower coracoid screw hole. It is again important to have an optimal view of the glenoid region to align the bone graft with the glenoid surface.

Tips and Tricks

It is important to hold the bone graft steady while implanting the upper screw, aided by the TCD. Once again, retractors have an essential function in the surgical procedure. The Fukuda retractor is kept in the lateral portion, the forked Hohmann-type retractor is used in the medial region, and a swan retractor is used for the upper portion of the subscapularis muscle.

Complications

- If the preceding steps have been performed correctly, no particular complications will be encountered.

Fig. 3.13a, b. **a** Two cannulated screws are inserted with the help of the two Kirschner wires. **b** The superior screw is inserted first. After the first screw, the temporary compression device is removed, maintaining the inferior Kirschner wire to insert the second screw

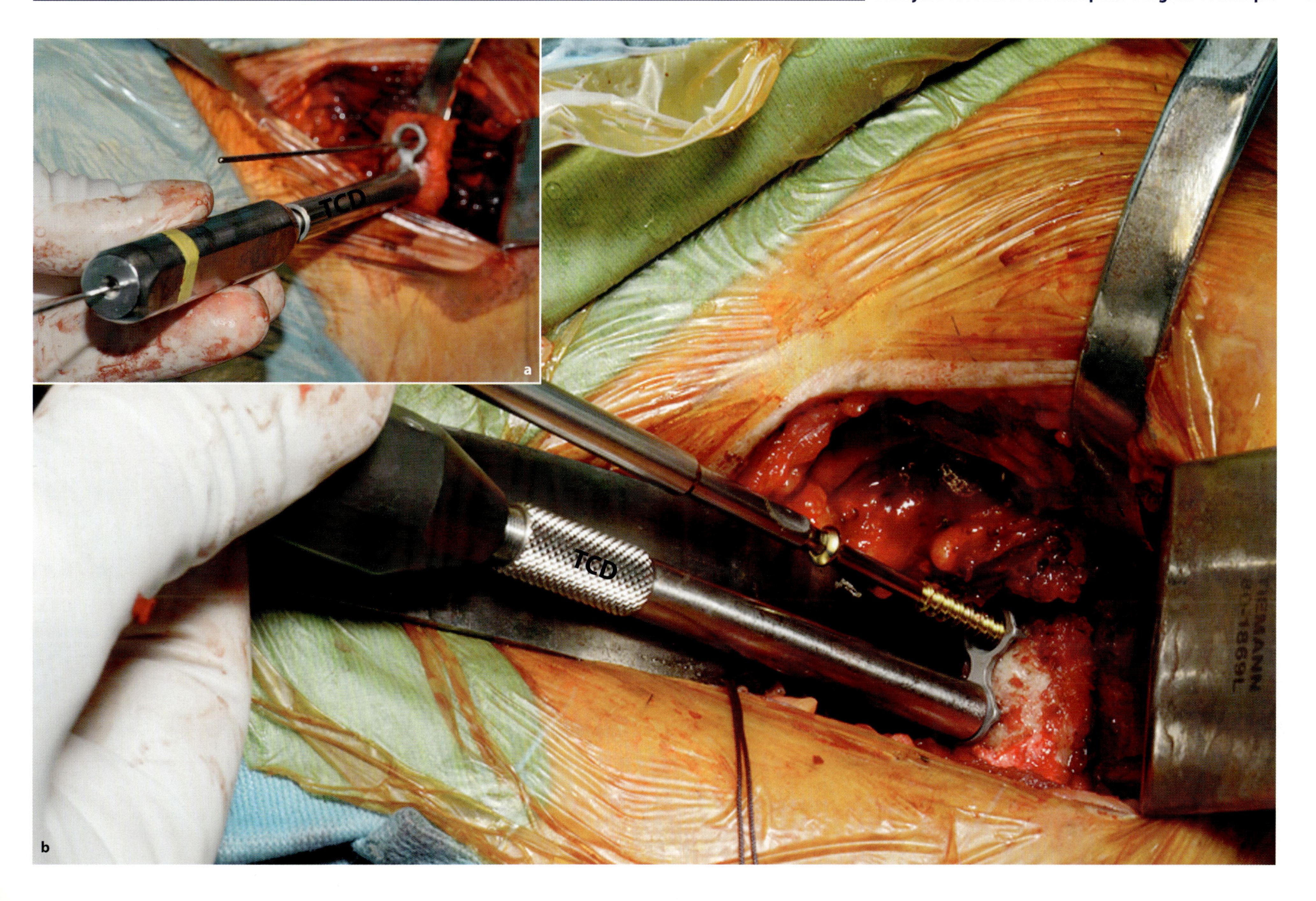
TCD
a
TCD
b

3.4.12 Final Result

Because of the medial wedge of the plate, the slight medial tilt will improve contact between screw head and plate (Fig. 3.14a-c). Both screws must engage the posterior cortex of the scapula. The Fukuda retractor is removed, and the arm is placed in abduction and external rotation. The capsule and subscapularis muscle is sutured laterally only but not reattached to the medial region from which they were detached. As the Latarjet procedure is effective [29, 30], we do not stress the need for capsular repair on the glenoid or capsular reinforcement. We perform a capsular repair only for patients with associated hyperlaxity.

The triple effect of the Latarjet procedure is thus be achieved, with the coracoid bone graft positioned in the anterior portion of the glenoid, the subscapularis muscle split, and conjoined tendon positioned astride the lower portion of the subscapularis. Given the effects of the Latarjet procedure, we do not see a need for capsular repair on the glenoid margin, a procedure that can lead to range of motion restrictions. Finally, the wound is closed in layers.

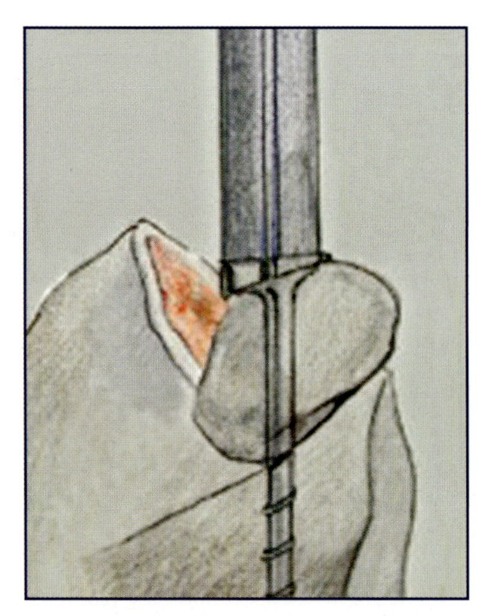

Positioning of bone graft on the glenoid neck in axial view

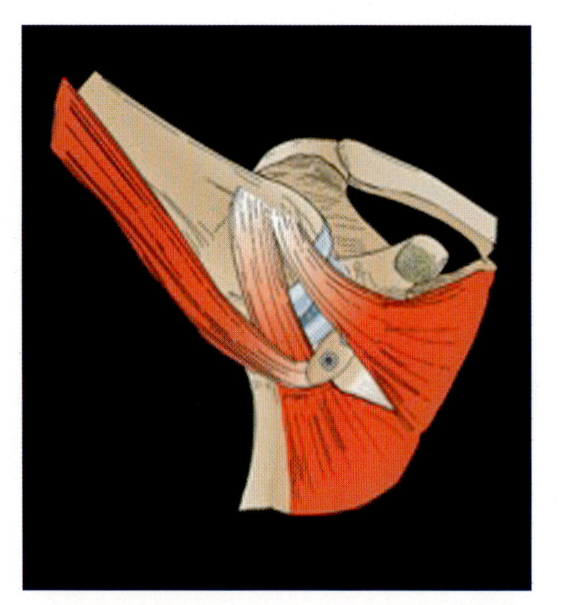

Final result of the Latarjet procedure in anterior view

Fig. 3.14a-c. **a** The two screws and plate are placed on the coracoid graft. The bone block will perfectly address the shape of the glenoid neck. **b** The lateral position of the graft is clearly in line with the glenoid surface

a
b
c

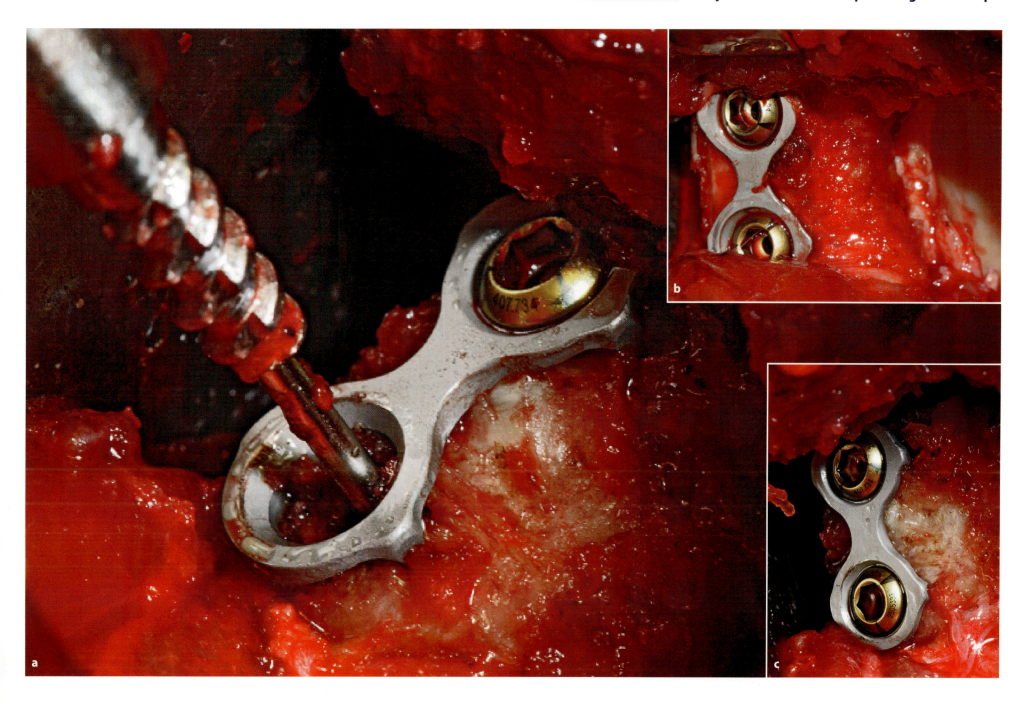

References

1. Latarjet M (1958) Technique of coracoid preglenoid arthroereisis in the treatment of recurrent dislocation of the shoulder. Lyon Chir 54:604-607 [article in French]
2. Yamamoto N, Itoi E, Hidekazu A et al (2007) Contact between the glenoid and the humeral head in abduction, external rotation, and horizontal extension: a new concept of glenoid track. J Shoulder Elbow Surg 16:649-656
3. Gill TJ, Micheli LJ, Gebhard F, Binder C (1997) Bankart repair for anterior instability of the shoulder. Long-term outcome. J Bone Joint Surg Am 79:850-857
4. Cole BJ, Warner JJ (2000) Arthroscopic versus open Bankart repair for traumatic anterior shoulder instability. Clin Sports Med 19:19-48
5. Rowe C, Patel D, Southmayd W (1978) The Bankart procedure: a long-term end-result study. J Bone Joint Surg Am 60:1-16
6. Helfet AJ (1958) Coracoid transplantation for recurring dislocation of the shoulder. J Bone Joint Surg Br 40:198-202
7. de Waal Malefijt J, Ooms AJ, van Rens TJ (1985) A comparison of the results of the Bristow-Latarjet procedure and the Bankart/Putti-Platt operation for recurrent anterior dislocation of the shoulder. Acta Orthop Belg 51:831-842
8. Rowe C, Zarins B, Ciullo J (1984) Recurrent anterior dislocation of the shoulder after surgical repair. Apparent causes of failure and treatment. J Bone Joint Surg Am 66:159-168
9. Hovelius L, Thorling J, Fredin H (1979) Recurrent anterior dislocation of the shoulder. Results after the Bankart and Putti-Platt operations. J Bone Joint Surg Am 61:566-569
10. McAuliffe TB, Pangayatselvan T, Bayley I (1988) Failed surgery for recurrent anterior dislocation of the shoulder. Causes and management. J Bone Joint Surg Br 70:798-801
11. Zabinski SJ, Callaway GH, Cohen S, Warren RF (1999) Revision shoulder stabilization: 2- to 10-year results. J Shoulder Elbow Surg 8:58-65
12. Young DC, Rockwood CA Jr (1991) Complications of a failed Bristow procedure and their management. J Bone Joint Surg Am 73:969-981
13. Jia X, Petersen SA, Khosravi AH et al (2009) Examination of the shoulder: the past, the present, and the future. J Bone Joint Surg Am 91(Suppl)6:10-18
14. Ticker JB, Warner JJ (2000) Selective capsular shift technique for anterior and anterior-inferior glenohumeral instability. Clin Sports Med 19:1-17
15. Neer CS 2nd (1985) Involuntary inferior and multidirectional instability of the shoulder: etiology, recognition, and treatment. Instr Course Lect 34:232-238
16. Faber K, Homa K, Hawkins R (1999) Translation of the glenohumeral joint in patients with anterior instability: awake examination versus examination with the patient under anesthesia. J Shoulder Elbow Surg 8:320-323
17. Speer KP, Hannafin JA, Altchek DW, Warren RF (1994) An evaluation of the shoulder relocation test. Am J Sports Med 22:177-183
18. Cofield RH, Irving JF (1987) Evaluation and classification of shoulder instability: with special reference to examination under anesthesia. Clin Orthop 223:32-43
19. Rockwood CA Jr, Jensen KL (1998) X-ray evaluation of shoulder problems. In: Rockwood CA Jr, Matsen FA 3rd, eds. The shoulder, 2nd edn. Saunders, Philadelphia, pp 199-231
20. Baudi P, Righi P, Bolognedi D et al (2005) How to identify and calculate glenoid bone deficit. Chir Organi Mov 90:145-152
21. Speer KP, Deng X, Borrero S et al (1994) Biomechanical evaluation of a simulated Bankart lesion. J Bone Joint Surg Am 76:1819-1826
22. Hubbell JD, Ahmad S, Bezenoff LS et al (2004) Comparison of shoulder stabilization using arthroscopic transglenoid sutures versus open capsulolabral repairs: a 5-year minimum follow-up. Am J Sports Med 32:650-654
23. Edwards TB, Walch G (2002) The Latarjet procedure for recurrent anterior shoulder instability: rationale and technique. Oper Tech Sports Med 10:25-32
24. Young AA, Maia R, Berhouet J, Walch G (2011) Open Latarjet procedure for management of bone loss in anterior instability of the glenohumeral joint. J Shoulder Elbow Surg 20(Suppl 2):S61-S69
25. Burkhart SS, De Beer JF (2000) Traumatic glenohumeral bone defects and their relationship to failure of arthroscopic Bankart repairs: significance of the inverted-pear glenoid and the humeral engaging Hill-Sachs lesion. Arthroscopy 16:677-694
26. Balg F, Boileau P (2007) The Instability Severity Index Score: a simple pre-operative score to select patients for arthroscopic or open shoulder stabilisation. J Bone Joint Surg Br 89:1470-1477
27. Clavert P, Lutz J-C, Wolfram-Gabel R et al (2009) Relationships of the musculocutaneous nerve and the coracobrachialis during coracoid abutment procedure (Latarjet procedure). Surg Radiol Anat 31:49-53

28. Di Giacomo G, Pouliart N, Costantini A, De Vita A (2008) Atlas of functional shoulder anatomy. Springer-Verlag, Milan
29. Clavert P, Kempf JF, Kahn JL (2009) Biomechanics of open Bankart and coracoid abutment procedures in a human cadaveric shoulder model. J Shoulder Elbow Surg 18: 69-74
30. Wellmann M, Petersen W, Zantop T et al (2009) Open shoulder repair of osseous glenoid defects. Biomechanical effectiveness of the Latarjet procedure versus a contoured structural bone graft. Am J Sports Med 37:87-94

Chapter 4 – Double-row Capsulolabral Repair

Craig S. Mauro, Sommer Hammoud, Courtney K. Dawson and David W. Altchek

4.1 Introduction

Both open and arthroscopic anterior shoulder stabilization procedures are commonly performed to address shoulder instability and have been shown to be successful in restoring shoulder stability and patient function. However, a critical review of the risk factors for recurrent instability following anterior stabilization is required to determine which patients may benefit from open stabilization, as recurrence rates following arthroscopic stabilization have historically been higher than with open stabilization. Multiple prospective studies have implicated younger patient age, capsular stretching, ligamentous laxity, contact athletics, and glenoid or humeral bone loss as risk factors for arthroscopic anterior shoulder stabilization failure [1–7].

The contact athlete is exposed to significant trauma and is thus particularly susceptible to recurrent instability after an initial arthroscopic stabilization [8–10]. Failure rates of stabilization procedures in contact athletes are reported to be higher than the general population [9–11]. Cho et al. compared collision and noncollision athletes who underwent arthroscopic stabilization for shoulder instability and found a recurrence rate of 28.6% in the collision group versus 6.7% in the noncollision group [9]. Rhee et al. compared arthroscopic and open anterior stabilization in 46 collision athletes and found a recurrence of 25% in the arthroscopic group versus 12.5% in the open group [10]. These high rates have led some to suggest that initial open stabilization may be more appropriate in the contact athlete. Pagnani and Dome reported that only 3% of their cohort of US football players developed postoperative subluxation after initial open stabilization [8]. These results indicate that open repair may offer certain advantages that arthroscopic techniques have not yet been able to duplicate in this population of high-demand contact athletes.

Many factors must be considered in determining which patients require surgical stabilization for anterior shoulder instability. Once a decision for surgery has been made, the surgeon must consider multiple patient-specific risk factors for recurrent instability in determining which stabilization approach to utilize. In this chapter, we present an overview of our evaluation and management algorithm of the patient with anterior shoulder instability. We then outline our rationale for electing an open stabilization and describe our technique.

4.2 Preoperative Evaluation

A detailed history that includes mechanism of instability, time from initial episode, number of dislocations, sports participation, and positions that reproduce symptoms is obtained. Physical examination of both shoulders includes measurement of range of motion in forward flexion, internal rotation behind the back, external rotation at the side, and internal and external rotation with the arm in 90° of abduction. Strength testing is performed using a five-point scale. The anterior apprehension test is performed with the patient in the supine position. The shoulder is abducted 90° and rotated externally until the point of apprehension. Anterior and posterior humeral translations, as well as inferior instability (sulcus sign), are also assessed. Grading of joint translation is as follows: grade 1, translation of the humeral head to the glenoid rim; grade 2, translation of the humeral head over the glenoid rim with spontaneous relocation; grade 3, translation of the humeral head over the glenoid rim with locking.

Patients with suspected shoulder instability upon history and physical examination are evaluated with anteroposterior radiographs in internal and external rotation, a scapular-Y, and axillary views to evaluate the glenoid shape and the presence of a bony Bankart or Hill-Sachs lesion. Magnetic resonance imaging (MRI) is critical for assessing the labrum and ruling out other intra-articular pathology prior to surgical intervention. In cases where bone loss is suspected, we perform a 3D computed tomography (CT) scan as part of the preoperative workup.

4.3 Treatment Algorithm

Every surgeon's approach depends heavily on the factors listed above and surgeon preference, experience, and comfort with more advanced arthroscopic and open techniques. Our treatment for anterior shoulder instability depends primarily on patient age, athletic demands, number of previous dislocations, and capsule, glenoid, and humeral head status. In most patients presenting with acute fractures of the glenoid or humeral avulsion of the glenohumeral ligament (HAGL), we recommend initial open treatment. All first-time dislocations undergo a trial of nonoperative treatment that includes a standardized physical therapy rehabilitation protocol and abduction bracing for selected at-risk contact athletics. Patients who fail nonoperative treatment and have recurrent instability that interferes with athletic activity or activities of daily life are considered for open or arthroscopic stabilization. We perform an arthroscopic anterior stabilization in the majority of cases, especially in patients who have lower athletic demands.

We generally recommend an open procedure for patients who participate in higher-level contact sports (football, wrestling, lacrosse) and those with poor-quality tissue, significant bone loss, multiple dislocations, and/or significant capsular laxity. We are also more inclined to recommend open stabilization in younger patients (age <20) with any of the other risk factors listed. In patients who failed initial arthroscopic anterior stabilization, we consider arthroscopic revision if failure of the index procedure was due to significant trauma and if the patient does not meet the other criteria described for open stabilization. Otherwise, we also recommend open stabilization in the revision setting, particularly in the presence of poor tissue quality.

In patients with bone loss, we tend to more readily recommend open stabilization. If the patient does not have the previously described risk factors for failure and has glenoid bone loss of up to 20% of the glenoid width, we perform arthroscopic stabilization. If bone loss is between 20% and 30%, we perform open stabilization of the capsulolabral complex and repair any concomitant bony Bankart lesion. With anterior glenoid bone loss >30%, we recommend open stabilization with the native glenoid fragment (if available) or with a glenoid augmentation, such with as a Latarjet procedure. Similarly, Hill-Sachs defects <20% can be treated with standard arthroscopic shoulder stabilization. Hill-Sachs lesions of 20–30% may require tendon transfer or bone grafting in an open fashion, whereas lesions >30% require consideration for osteochondral allograft transplantation.

The open stabilization technique we utilize, which we describe in detail in this chapter, is a double-row capsulolabral repair. This technique is similar to that previously described by Ahmad et al. and Lafosse et al. [12, 13] and serves to reinforce the repair of the capsulolabral complex back to the anterior and medial glenoid neck. It can be utilized in patients who present in a complex revision setting or who meet our described criteria for open stabilization.

4.4 Surgical Technique

Typically, a regional interscalene block is performed; general anesthesia is acceptable and allows contralateral shoulder examination. The patient is positioned in the modified beach-chair configuration using a full-length beanbag on an adjustable operating-room table. The bag is carefully molded and positioned on the table to provide access to the medial aspect of the scapula. An adjustable arm holder is utilized for positioning the arm and shoulder during the procedure. Examination under anesthesia of the affected shoulder is performed. Shoulder range of motion, anterior and posterior humeral head translation (Fig. 4.1), and sulcus sign (Fig. 4.2) are assessed and documented.

Fig. 4.1. Anterior and posterior humeral head translation is assessed and graded as follows: grade 1, translation of the humeral head to the glenoid rim; grade 2, translation of the humeral head over the glenoid rim with spontaneous relocation; grade 3, translation of the humeral head over the glenoid rim with locking

Fig. 4.2. Sulcus sign, which helps identifying inferior or multidirectional instability, is a measure of the gap that appears beneath the acromion. With the patient's arm at the side, the examiner stabilizes the acromion with one hand while applying traction to the humerus with the other

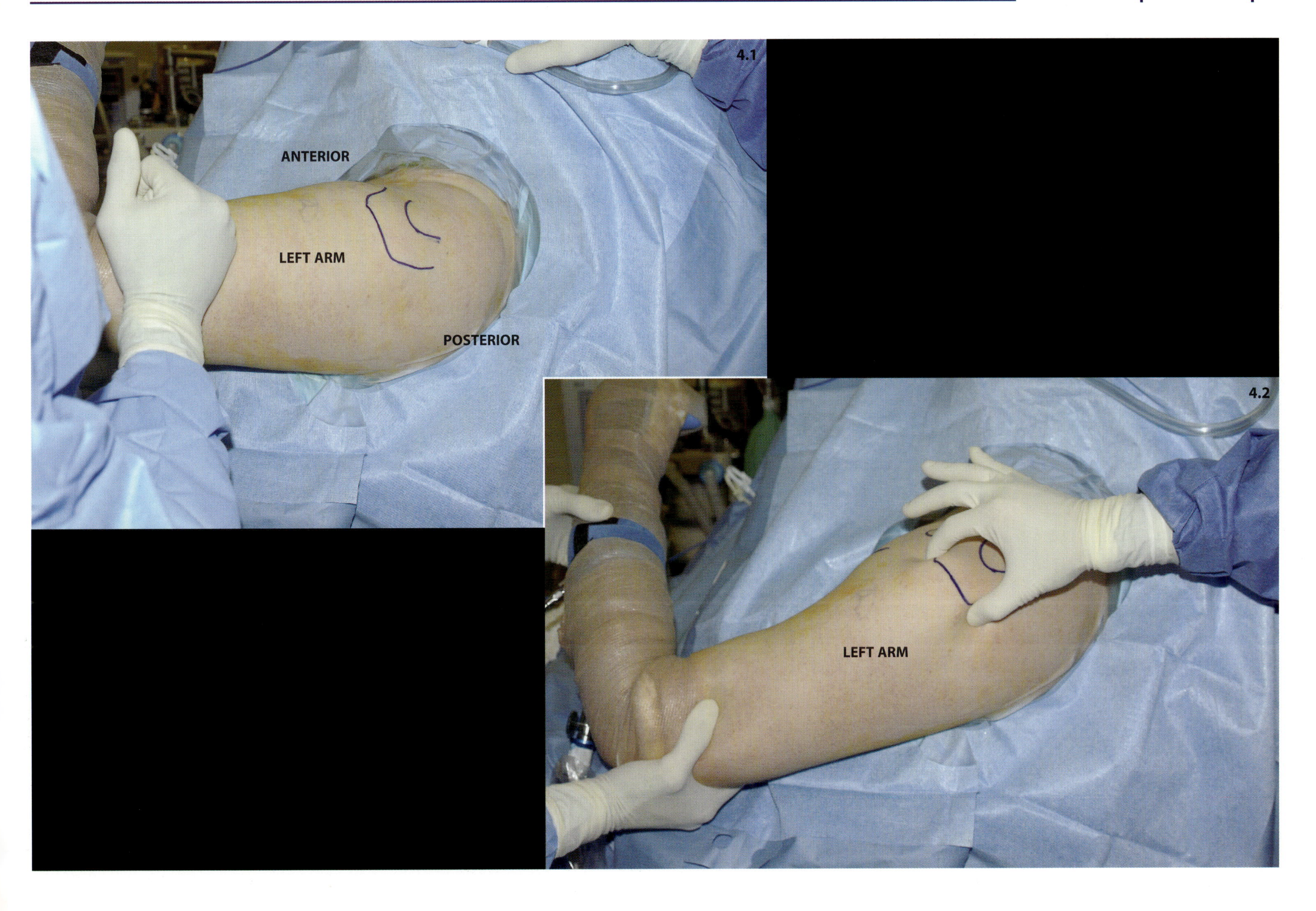
4.1
ANTERIOR
LEFT ARM
POSTERIOR
4.2
LEFT ARM

A standard posterior arthroscopic portal is established, and a systematic, diagnostic examination of the glenohumeral joint is performed. Labral lesions, glenoid deficits, Hill-Sachs defects, and capsular tissue quality are evaluated.

A deltopectoral approach is performed using a longitudinal incision extending proximally from the axillary crease (Fig. 4.3). Meticulous hemostasis and thick flaps are established. The cephalic vein (Fig. 4.4) is mobilized laterally, and the interval between deltoid and pectoralis major is established. The clavipectoral fascia is incised just lateral to the conjoined tendon, and a self-retaining retractor is placed beneath the conjoined tendon medially and the deltoid muscle laterally. The anterior humeral

Fig. 4.3. Longitudinal incision extending superiorly from the axillary crease

Fig. 4.4. Fat stripe is identified over the cephalic vein

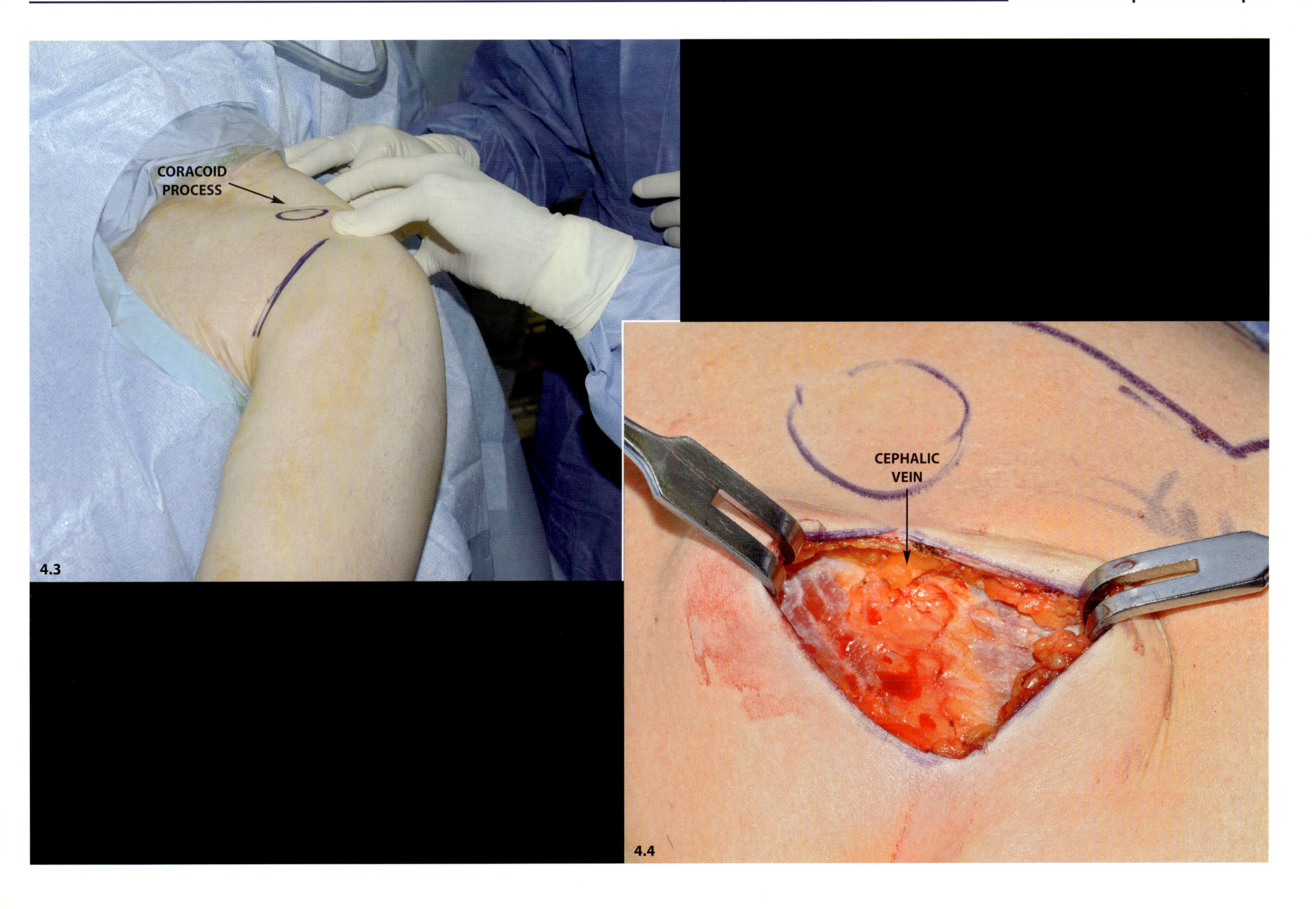
CORACOID
PROCESS
4.3
CEPHALIC
VEIN
4.4

circumflex vessels at the lower border of the subscapularis muscle are coagulated (Fig. 4.5).

Managing the subscapularis tendon and anterior capsule is a critical portion of the case, as the plane between the subscapularis tendon and the anterior portion of the capsule must be developed. To establish this plane, the subscapularis must first be reflected (Fig. 4.6). This step can be achieved in one of several ways. In the first method, the inferior, more muscular, portion of the subscapularis may be split in line with the fibers. A large, curved Kelly clamp is then placed through this split from inferior to superior in the plane deep to the subscapularis and superficial to the anterior capsule. A knife is then used to divide the tendon over the Kelly clamp, taking care to leave a stump of tendon on the humeral side for later repair. The subscapularis tendon is tagged with suture and reflected medially.

A second method of tagging and reflecting the subscapularis involves simply obliquely dividing the subscapularis tendon, again leaving a stump on the humeral side for later repair. The tissue is carefully evaluated, as it is divided layer by layer to ensure that the capsule is not violated. The subscapularis is tagged and reflected medially (Fig. 4.6).

A final method that may be employed involves simply incising and reflecting the subscapularis tendon and the capsule from the humerus in one layer. The position of this split is, as with the other techniques, medial enough within the substance of the subscapularis tendon that a stump of tissue repair remains in place for later repair. Once they are freed, the interval between the subscapularis tendon and the capsule can be developed in a similar fashion to the other techniques.

The medial flap of the subscapularis is dissected from the anterior part of the capsule medially to the glenoid margin and inferiorly to the 6 o'clock position. The capsule is thoroughly inspected. Redundancy of the anterior and inferior portions of the capsule is obvious at this point. Also, any capsular tears or rotator interval defects should be appreciated.

Fig. 4.5. Anterior humeral circumflex vessels at the lower border of the subscapularis muscle are coagulated and the anticipated subscapularis tenotomy is defined

Fig. 4.6. Subscapularis tendon is tagged with suture and reflected medially after cutting. Medial flap of subscapularis is dissected from the anterior part of the capsule

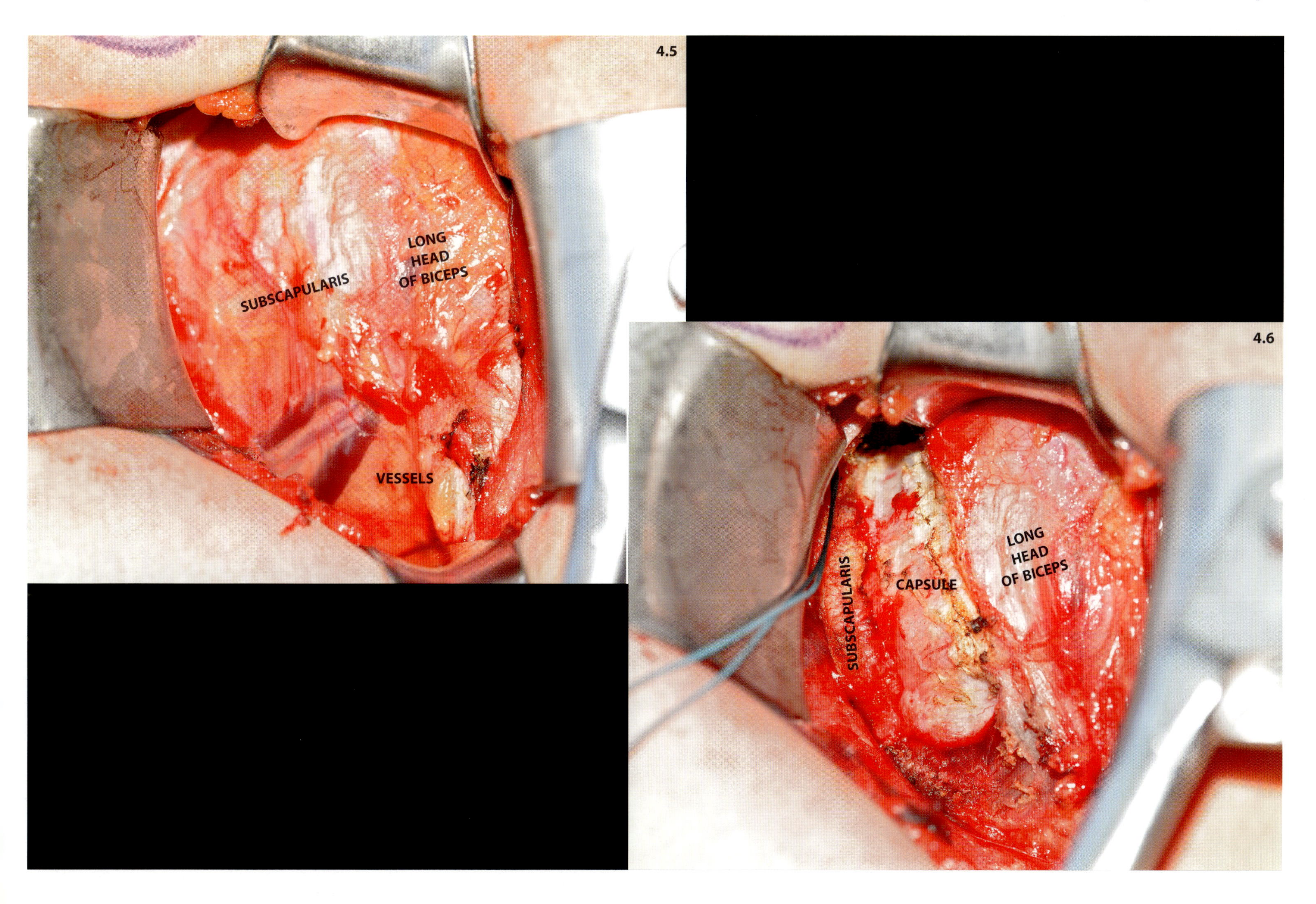
4.5
LONG
HEAD
OF BICEPS
SUBSCAPULARIS
VESSELS
4.6
LONG
HEAD
OF BICEPS
CAPSULE
SUBSCAPULARIS

If not already created with the subscapularis release, a longitudinal incision along the humeral attachment of the capsule is made (Fig. 4.7). The capsule is tagged while it is released from the superior to the inferior-most portion of the humerus. External rotation of the humerus facilitates the exposure. Special care is taken to protect the axillary nerve during this portion of the procedure. This incision allows for further inspection of the joint and assessment of capsular mobility and redundancy. A finger may be placed into the joint, and while tension is applied to the tagged anterior portion of the capsule, tension of the posterior inferior glenohumeral ligament is assessed.

A Fukuda humeral head retractor is placed into the shoulder joint, posterior to the glenoid, and is used to retract the humeral head posteriorly to expose the glenoid. A pitchfork retractor is placed medially, within the subscapularis fossa, to facilitate inspection of the anteroinferior capsulolabral complex (Fig. 4.8). The

Fig. 4.7. Longitudinal incision along the humeral attachment of the capsule. Laxity is evaluated

Fig. 4.8. Inspection of the anterior-inferior glenoid demonstrates evidence of a previous labral repair and a medially scarred capsulolabral complex

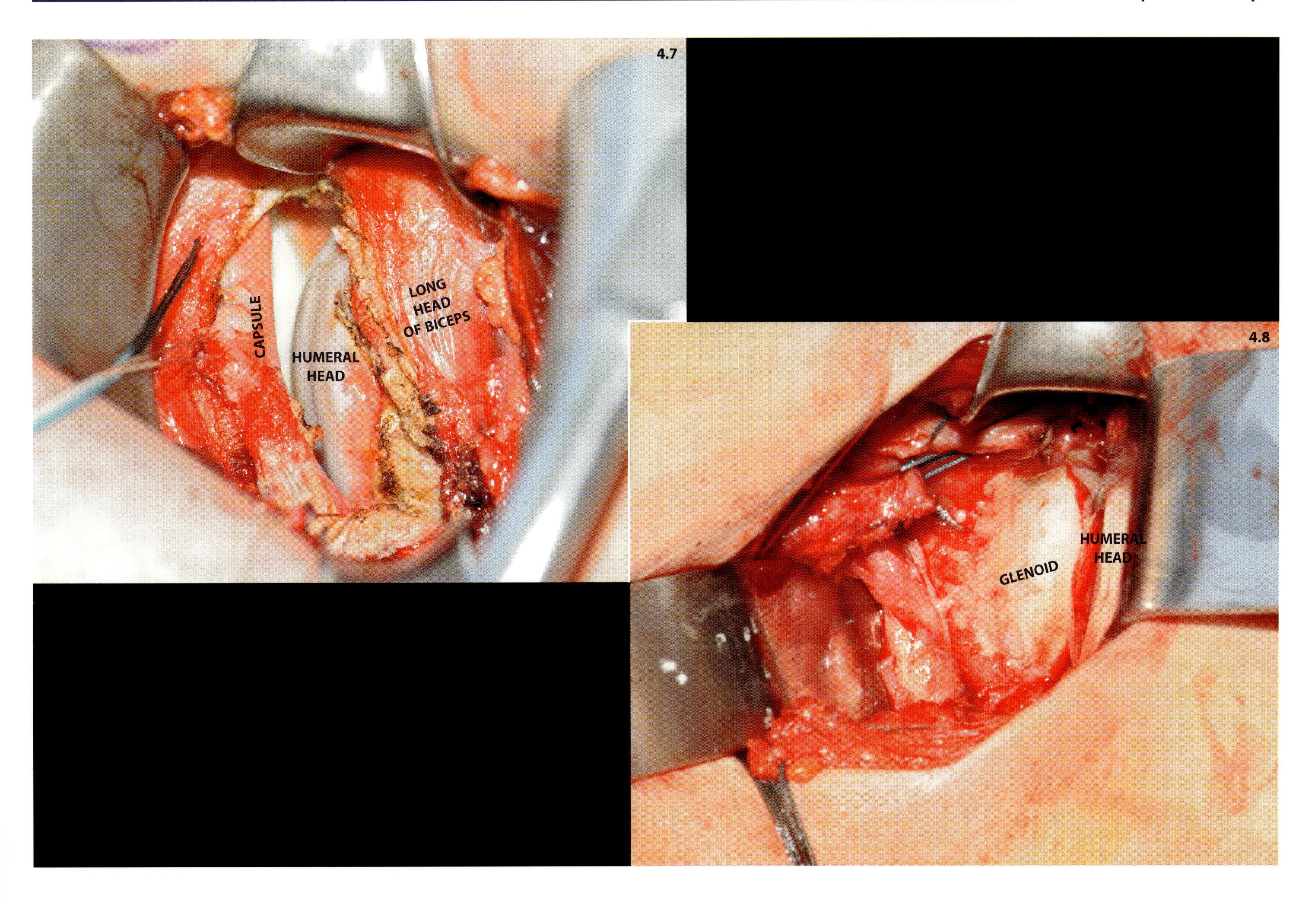
4.7
CAPSULE
HUMERAL HEAD
LONG HEAD OF BICEPS
4.8
GLENOID
HUMERAL HEAD

anteromedial glenoid is then exposed by elevating the capsulolabral complex off the underlying bony surface of the anterior glenoid neck. To perform this release, an elevator is placed between the labrum and the glenoid and manipulated to ensure that the anterior glenoid neck is completely exposed. The pitchfork retractor is then placed deep to the labrum to completely expose the glenoid neck (Fig. 4.9).

A hole for a 3.0-mm Bio-SutureTak (Arthrex, Naples, FL, USA) suture anchor is drilled in the glenoid neck at a point 1 cm medial to the edge of the glenoid articular surface at the 5:30 position. The anchor is then placed. A second suture anchor is placed at the 4:30 position and also 1 cm medial to the edge of the glenoid articular surface (Fig. 4.10). The pitchfork retractor is removed and placed deep to the subscapularis and outside the capsule. Both limbs of the

Fig. 4.9. Glenoid neck is then exposed by elevating the capsulolabral complex off the underlying bony surface

Fig. 4.10. Two medial anchors are placed in the glenoid neck

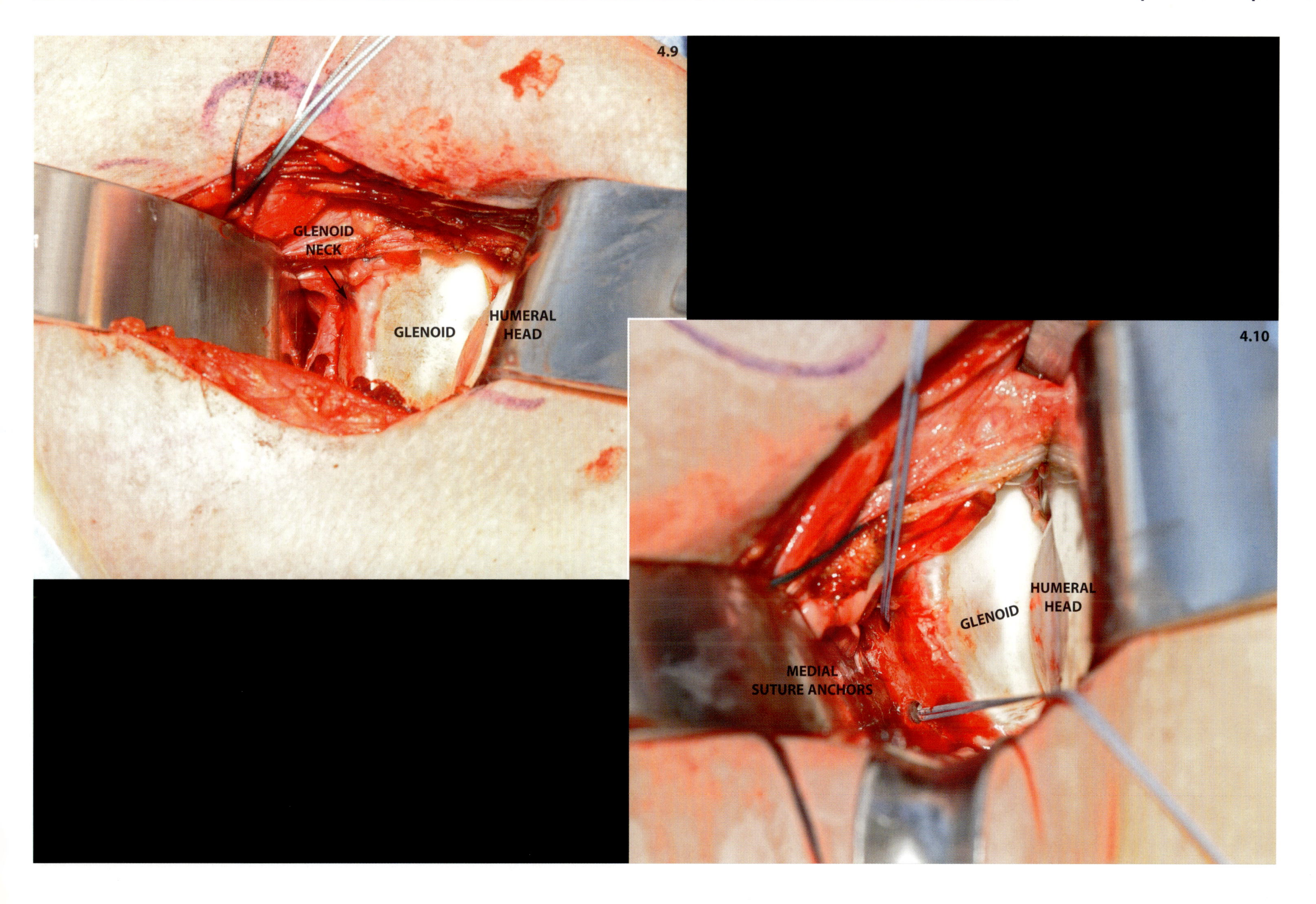
4.9
GLENOID
NECK
GLENOID
HUMERAL
HEAD
4.10
HUMERAL
HEAD
GLENOID
MEDIAL
SUTURE ANCHORS

suture from both suture anchors are then sequentially passed with a free needle through the adjacent capsulolabral tissue, allowing for any necessary lateral advancement of the capsulolabral complex. The sutures are retrieved and held outside the capsule (Fig. 4.11). No knots are tied at this point. Holes for 2.9-mm PEEK PushLock (Arthrex) anchors are then drilled on the edge of the glenoid articular surface at the 5:30 and 4:30 positions (Fig. 4.12). The suture limbs from the inferior medial suture anchor are loaded into the first PushLock. Tension is applied to the sutures, and the PushLock is impacted into the inferior hole with a mallet. This process is

Fig. 4.11. Sutures from both anchors are passed through the medial capsulolabral complex

Fig. 4.12. Suture limbs are loaded, and the PushLock is impacted into the hole on the edge of the glenoid articular surface

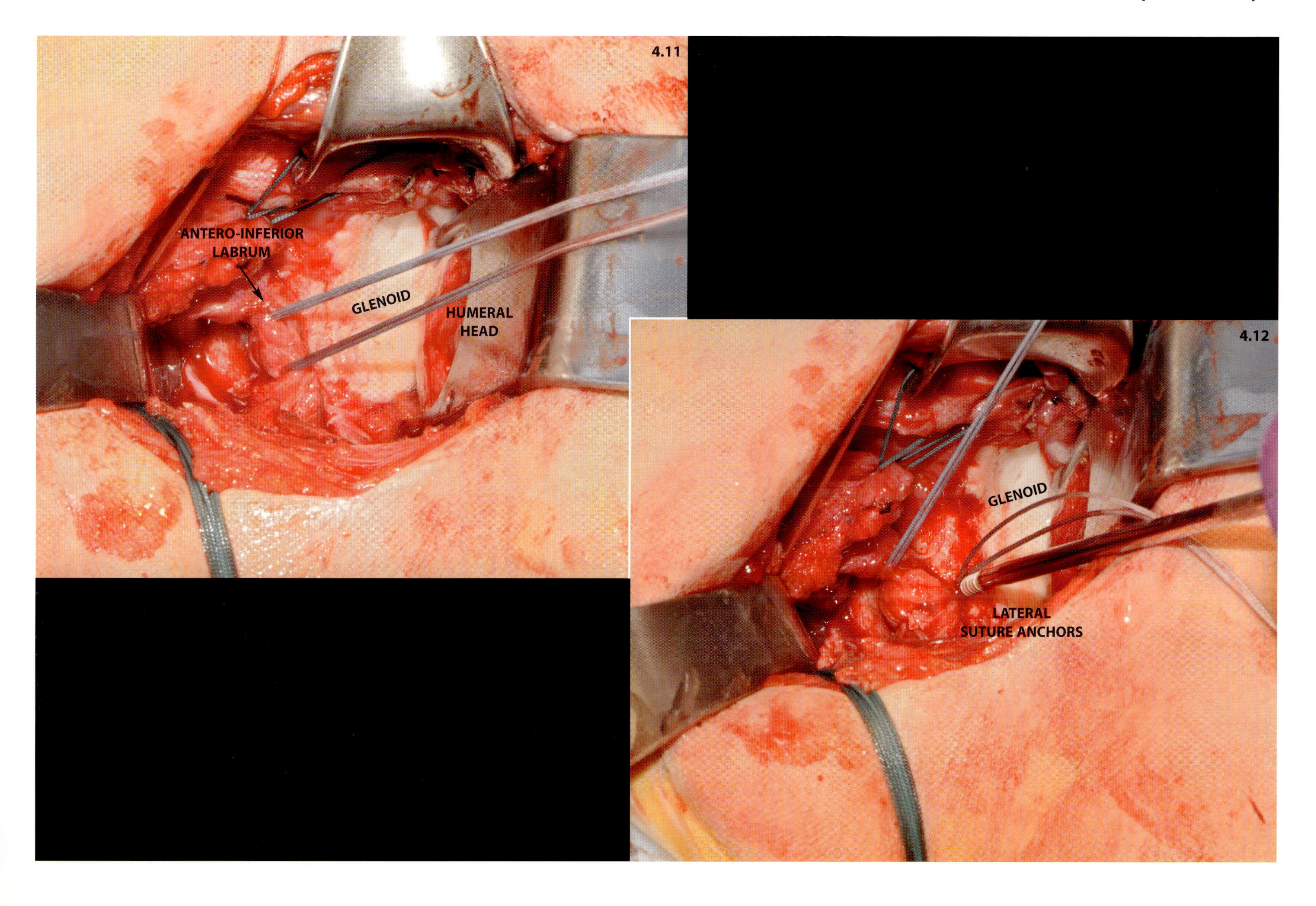
4.11
ANTERO-INFERIOR
LABRUM
GLENOID
HUMERAL
HEAD
4.12
GLENOID
LATERAL
SUTURE ANCHORS

repeated for the sutures from the superior suture anchor to complete the repair (Fig 4.13).

This double-row capsulolabral repair may be performed with or without a capsular shift. If there is very redundant capsule, a lateral capsular shift is performed. A second capsular incision, transverse and at the level of the mid glenoid, is then made. This second incision thereby creates two flaps in the capsule: one inferior and one superior. The inferior flap will be mobilized superiorly and laterally and the superior flap inferiorly and laterally. Four double-loaded anchors are placed from inferior to superior in the anatomic neck of the humerus. Close attention must be paid to managing the sutures, as numerous sutures remain in the surgical field once the anchors have been placed.

The shoulder and arm are placed in position in preparation for the capsular shift. The shoulder is placed in about 30° of forward flexion to allow the humeral head to fall back into a reduced position on the glenoid. The arm is then placed in 45° of abduction and 30–45° of external rotation. The degree of external rotation is dependent of the patient. Overhead-throwing athletes are stabilized with the shoulder in more external rotation to allow for recovery of motion required for throwing.

The capsular shift of the inferior flap is performed first. This flap is advanced superiorly and laterally to eliminate inferior capsular laxity to a point where the desired, previously established, external rotation is still just possible. Sutures from the most inferior anchor are passed through the capsular tissue in a horizontal mattress-stitch fashion to maintain the capsule in this position. The sutures are tagged for later tying (Fig. 4.14). Sutures from the more superior anchors are sequentially passed through the inferior flap to advance and secure it back to the humerus. The inferior flap, when advanced, usually covers the entire defect created from both flaps. Once the sutures have been passed through the inferior flap (usually from the inferior two to three anchors), they are sequentially tied down on the humerus from inferior to superior. The needles are maintained on the sutures for subsequent reattachment of the superior flap. The rotator interval is closed by stitching the top portion of the inferior flap superiorly to the rotator interval tissue with interrupted no. 2 nonabsorbable sutures.

The superior flap is advanced inferiorly and laterally over the inferior flap. Sutures from the previously placed superior two to three anchors are passed through the lateral portion of the superior flap in a horizontal mattress-stitch fashion. Once all sutures have been passed, they are tied down from superior to inferior. The overlapping inferior margin of the superior flap is also repaired to the inferior flap with interrupted no. 2 nonabsorbable sutures. The repair is then evaluated. The humeral head should be centered on the glenoid. Posterior instability should be reduced, and inferior and anterior instability should be eliminated. External rotation should be at least 30–40° without undue tension on the repair.

Attention is then turned to the subscapularis tendon repair. With the shoulder still in the slightly externally rotated position, the tendon ends are brought together to restore the anatomic

Fig. 4.13. Completed double-row repair

Fig. 4.14. Lateral capsule is restored with inferior-to-superior shift to reduce inferior capsular laxity to the desired point, with the arm in external rotation

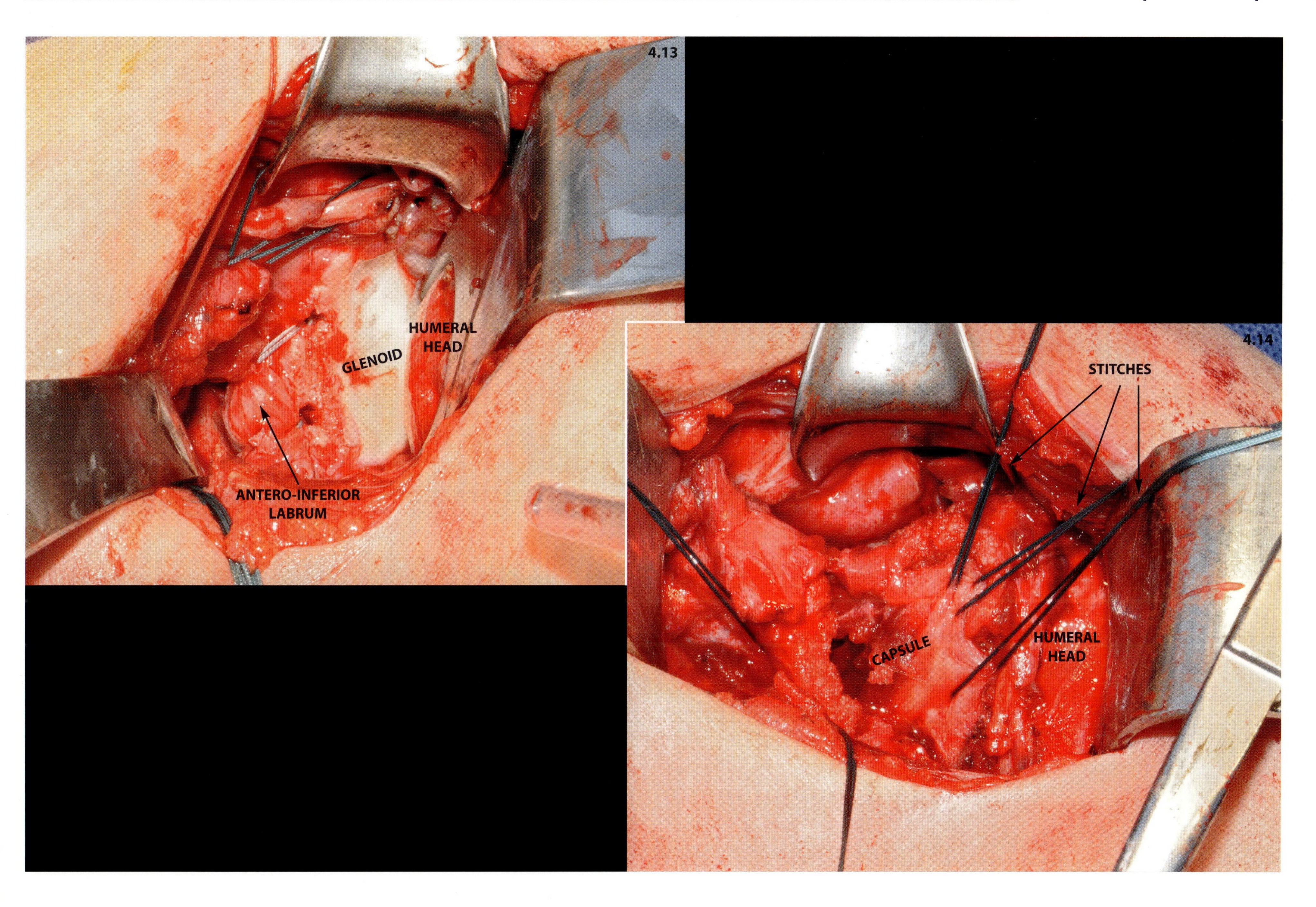
4.13
HUMERAL HEAD
GLENOID
ANTERO-INFERIOR LABRUM
4.14
STITCHES
CAPSULE
HUMERAL HEAD

length (Fig. 4.15). They are repaired from side to side with multiple interrupted figure-of-eight stitches using no. 2 nonabsorbable sutures (Fig. 4.16). The wound is closed over a suction drain. A shoulder immobilizer with an abduction pillow is worn to support the arm with the shoulder in neutral rotation and slight forward flexion and abduction.

4.5 Postoperative Rehabilitation

During the first 3 weeks, the goals of therapy are to promote healing and reduce pain, inflammation, and swelling. An independent home exercise program is prescribed that allows active-assisted range of motion (AAROM), including elevation in plane of scapula to 90°, external rotation to between 0 and 30°, scapular mobility and stability (side-lying, progressing to manual resistance), submaximal deltoid isometrics in neutral, and modalities for pain and edema.

During weeks 3–6, the goals of therapy are healing continuation and initiating restoration of scapular and rotator cuff strength. The immobilizer is discontinued between 4 and 6 weeks postoperatively. The patient continues with elevation to 145° and external rotation to 60°, scapular stabilization, and submaximal isometric internal and external rotation. Special care is taken to avoid excessive stretch to the anterior capsule and avoid rotator cuff inflammation.

During weeks 6–12, goals are to restore normal shoulder range of motion, strength, flexibility, and scapulohumeral rhythm. Restoration of upper extremity endurance is also initiated. The therapist should initiate AAROM in internal rotation, progress with isotonic and stabilization exercises for periscapular and rotator cuff muscles, and continue humeral head rhythmic stabilization.

During weeks 14–18, goals are to restore normal neuromuscular function, maintain strength and flexibility, restore isokinetic internal and external rotation strength at least equal to the unaffected side, and achieve a >66% isokinetic external-to-internal strength ratio. The therapist should employ full upper-extremity strengthening, external and internal rotation in the 90/90 position (overhead athlete), plyometrics, and a sport-activity-related program.

4.6 Conclusion

In the patient with anterior shoulder instability, addressing confounding factors such as bone loss, age, sport played, ligamentous laxity, capsule attenuation, and previous surgical approach employed is critical. We consider the open double-row capsulolabral repair described in certain high-risk populations, including younger patients, contact athletes, patients with mild bone loss on the glenoid or humerus, and patients with previous failed anterior stabilization. Further clinical evaluation of this emerging technique is warranted, as this improved restoration of the native capsulolabral anatomy may prove to decrease the rate of failed anterior shoulder stabilization, especially in high-risk patients.

Fig. 4.15. With the shoulder still in the slightly externally rotated position, tendon ends are brought together to restore anatomic length

Fig. 4.16. Subscapularis tendon ends are repaired from side to side with multiple interrupted figure-of-eight stitches using no. 2 nonabsorbable sutures

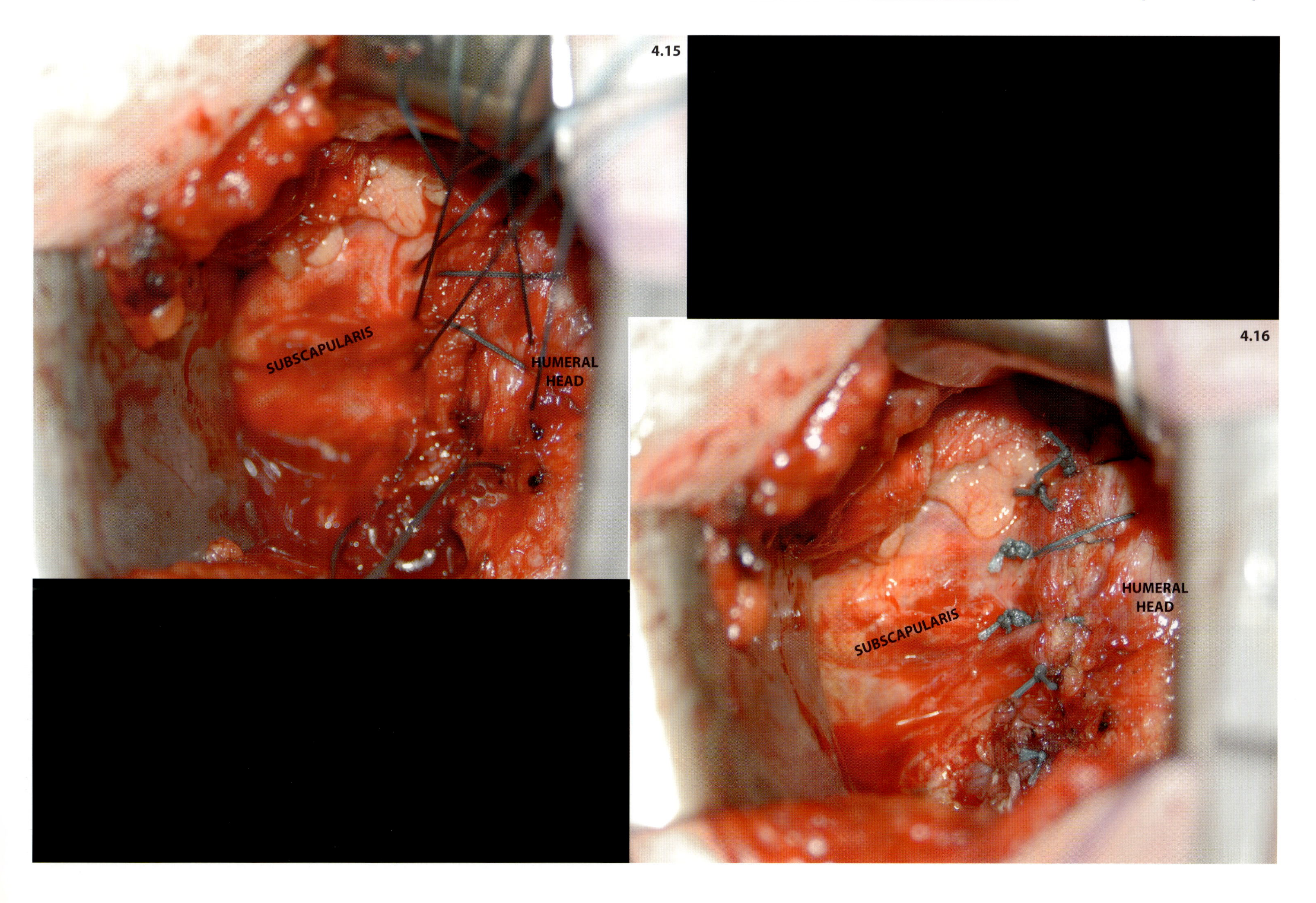
4.15
SUBSCAPULARIS
HUMERAL
HEAD
4.16
HUMERAL
HEAD
SUBSCAPULARIS

References

1. Voos JE, Livermore RW, Feeley BT et al (2009) Prospective evaluation of arthroscopic Bankart repairs for anterior instability. Am J Sports Med 38:302-307
2. Boileau P, Villalba M, Hery JY et al (2006) Risk factors for recurrence of shoulder instability after arthroscopic Bankart repair. J Bone Joint Surg Am 88:1755-1763
3. Burkhart SS, Danaceau SM (2000) Articular arc length mismatch as a cause of failed bankart repair. Arthroscopy 16:740-744
4. Burkhart SS, De Beer JF (2000) Traumatic glenohumeral bone defects and their relationship to failure of arthroscopic Bankart repairs: significance of the inverted-pear glenoid and the humeral engaging Hill-Sachs lesion. Arthroscopy 16:677-694
5. Rowe CR, Zarins B, Ciullo JV (1984) Recurrent anterior dislocation of the shoulder after surgical repair. Apparent causes of failure and treatment. J Bone Joint Surg Am 66:159-168
6. Bigliani LU, Newton PM, Steinmann SP et al (1998) Glenoid rim lesions associated with recurrent anterior dislocation of the shoulder. Am J Sports Med 26:41-45
7. Balg F, Boileau P (2007) The instability severity index score. A simple pre-operative score to select patients for arthroscopic or open shoulder stabilisation. J Bone Joint Surg Br 89:1470-1477
8. Pagnani MJ, Dome DC (2002) Surgical treatment of traumatic anterior shoulder instability in american football players. J Bone Joint Surg Am 84:711-715
9. Cho NS, Hwang JC, Rhee YG (2006) Arthroscopic stabilization in anterior shoulder instability: collision athletes versus noncollision athletes. Arthroscopy 22:947-953
10. Rhee YG, Ha JH, Cho NS (2006) Anterior shoulder stabilization in collision athletes: arthroscopic versus open Bankart repair. Am J Sports Med 34:979-985
11. Tauber M, Resch H, Forstner R et al (2004) Reasons for failure after surgical repair of anterior shoulder instability. J Shoulder Elbow Surg 13:279-285
12. Ahmad CS, Galano GJ, Vorys GC et al (2009) Evaluation of glenoid capsulolabral complex insertional anatomy and restoration with single- and double-row capsulolabral repairs. J Shoulder Elbow Surg 18:948-954
13. Lafosse L, Baier GP, Jost B (2006) Footprint fixation for arthroscopic reconstruction in anterior shoulder instability: the Cassiopeia double-row technique. Arthroscopy 22:231 e231-231, e236

Chapter 5 – The J-bone Graft for Anatomical Reconstruction of Glenoid Defects

Alexander Auffarth, Mark Tauber and Herbert Resch

5.1 Introduction

5.1.1 Classification of Instabilities

As with all challenges in medicine, the first step in treating shoulder instabilities is to define the problem. For this purpose, classifications have proven useful at the beginning of an individual treatment. In cases of shoulder dislocation, a feasible classification for use in clinical practice was introduced by Gerber and Nyffeler [1]. First, the surgeon must distinguish between static and dynamic instabilities. Static instabilities are rare compared with dynamic instabilities, and they can be asymptomatic; their treatment is not further discussed in this chapter. A dynamic instability is always initially caused by either one major trauma or recurrent minor traumas, and when diagnosed, it must be differentiated between six subgroups:

- chronic locked dislocation;
- unidirectional instability with or without hyperlaxity;
- multidirectional instability with or without hyperlaxity;
- voluntary instability.

Among them, cases with unidirectional instability with or without hyperlaxity are seen most frequently. These can, again, be subclassified into cases with anteroinferior instabilities and those with posterior instabilities. In our experience, unidirectional instability with hyperlaxity is more often associated with labral lesions than with osseous glenoid-rim defects. With respect to this classification, it is the unidirectional anteroinferior shoulder dislocation, most often without hyperlaxity, that is treated by the J-bone graft when it is accompanied by a relevant bone defect of the glenoid rim.

5.2 General Indications for Treating Shoulder Instability with Conservative and Surgical Techniques

Not all cases of shoulder dislocation require a bone graft procedure or, in fact, any other form of surgical treatment. Thus, when deciding between conservative and surgical treatment, the history of the patient's symptoms must be accurately evaluated. The first question to address is whether the current event is a first-time occurrence or a recurrent shoulder dislocation. Next, direction of the dislocation, e.g., anterior or posterior, should be determined, and the joint must be reduced after a primary radiograph is obtained. In cases of anterior dislocation, the joint is reduced using the technique preferred by the individual physician. With anterior dislocations, anesthesia is seldom necessary for reduction. When the shoulder is posteriorly dislocated, however, the joint is always reduced under general anesthesia. After successful joint reduction, a second radiograph is obtained. If neither the first nor the second radiograph shows an osseous lesion of the glenoid rim, the patient is treated conservatively, with the affected arm placed in a sling. In patients <60 years, the sling is used for 3 weeks, whereas it is removed after 1 week in older patients. In cases involving an osseous lesion at the glenoid rim, an arthroscopic screw fixation for large bone fragments and an open fixation for small fragments is our treatment of choice in younger patients. In older patients, only large fragments are fixed, whereas smaller osseous lesions are not directly addressed but treated by an open Latarjet procedure.

In contrast, when a patient is first seen with recurrent shoulder dislocations, many more influencing factors need to be taken into account to determine the treatment that best suits the case. In anamnesis, the onset of instability must be defined, especially following a subjectively traumatic or atraumatic event. Referring to the above classification system, there is no true atraumatic dynamic instability, but in the absence of a major single trauma, the event may be rated as such by the patient. This would most likely occur if repetitive microtraumas do not represent memorable events. Apart from this, the number of dislocations or subluxations should be evaluated. Furthermore, the surgeon must investigate which motions usually provoke dislocation in the individual patient. If the relevant injury always occurs during a sport, for example, this must be determined; if it occurs during sleep or activities of daily living, this must be evaluated as well. Next, the patient should be asked how the joint is usually reduced. This ensures that information will be recorded as to whether the patient has subluxations only with a trend toward spontaneous reduction, recurrent dislocations with the ability for self-reduction, or requires reduction by a physician. This history can be helpful for distinguishing between shoulders with or without hyperlaxity. The following physical examination should include the apprehension test, the reverse apprehension test, the relocation test, and laxity tests, such as the sulcus sign and anteroposterior translation.

Depending on the results of this investigation, patients can be assigned to one of the six subgroups mentioned above. Among patients with multidirectional instability and hyperlaxity and those with voluntary dislocations, treatment should be conservative, whereas the remaining patients should most likely be treated by surgery.

5.3 Algorithm and Indications for Determining Surgery Type and Timing

Of the remaining four types of dynamic instabilities, the locked dislocation is always treated by open reduction. Glenoid-rim fractures are not often seen in such cases. When a recurrent posttraumatic anterior shoulder dislocation is to be addressed, it will most often be unidirectional instability without hyperlaxity. Some patients will show signs of hyperlaxity; even fewer will have a multidirectional, unstable condition without hyperlaxity. In treating all three types, the surgeon must first distinguish between cases with soft tissue lesions only and those with osseous glenoid-rim defects. Prior to a surgical procedure, be it a primary stabilization or revision surgery for failed stabilization, a computed tomography (CT) scan of the injured shoulder should be obtained to assess the extent of glenoid damage and demonstrate indication for the bone-block procedure. For this purpose, a three-dimensional reconstruction of the glenoid provides the most accurate information. If a small osseous lesion is found, imaging of a soft tissue Bankart lesion by magnetic resonance imaging (MRI), for example, is considered dispensable. In such cases, arthroscopy is the treatment of choice and will show concomitant soft tissue lesions. Cases with narrow osseous lesions of the anteroinferior glenoid rim have been treated successfully with an arthroscopic technique [2]. In the presence of a relevant bony defect, however, a soft tissue procedure alone will most likely lead to postoperative recurrent dislocations. In this context, correlation between the extent of glenoid bone loss and loss of dislocation resistance has been demonstrated [1–5]. The larger an osseous defect at the glenoid rim, the more likely recurrent dislocations will occur.

In this context, a recent study recorded recurrence rates of 36% following arthroscopic soft tissue repairs after an average follow-up of 9 years in a series of 81 patients [6]. Among this population, it has not been sufficiently evaluated whether arthroscopic treatment is appropriate, given the coexistent osseous lesions or hyperlaxity. Thus, patients must be carefully assigned to either a soft tissue or osseous repair because the condition of the bony glenoid rim, on one hand, and hyperlaxity and number of dislocations, on the other, can determine the expected outcome of each procedure.

As an alternative, an open Bankart procedure can be performed. The open Bankart repair is now rarely performed in our practice. In our experience, for almost all cases, sufficient stabilization can be achieved by either an arthroscopic repair or the open J-bone graft [7], depending on the condition of the bony rim. Alternatively, a Neer T-shift procedure might be considered in cases of extensive hyperlaxity without an osseous glenoid-rim lesion. This may allow reinforcement of a thin anterior capsule by doubling it. Moreover, in the absence of a bony defect, another indication for open soft tissue repair might be an unstable shoulder with many previous dislocations that is threatening to dislocate with the arm just above the shoulder level.

In summary, we saw that 50% of all failed arthroscopic soft tissue repairs had bony-rim defects that had been not taken into account at the primary surgical repair [8]. Others report similar findings. An intact bony glenoid is required to reach the full range of motion of the shoulder joint [1, 4]. According to our regimen, soft tissue repair alone can only be performed in patients with a bony defect that does not exceed the width of the rim cortex.

5.4 Indications for the Authors' Technique

The classic indication for the J-bone-graft procedure is the recurrent dislocation with an anteroinferior bone defect of the glenoid exceeding the width of the rim cortex in a young, active patient. This procedure has shown promising results for preventing recurrent posttraumatic anterior shoulder dislocation with osseous glenoid defects in patients <60 years. Apart from these indications, the technique is used for revision stabilization after failed arthroscopic or open procedures. The primary surgical objective of this method is to reconstruct the anteroinferior glenoid surface to prevent further shoulder dislocations. Technical details and modifications of the former approach [7] are presented later in this chapter.

5.5 Contraindications

Contraindications for the J-bone-graft technique include recurrent anterior shoulder dislocations without a glenoid rim defect. The procedure may not be suitable for patients >60 years because of an assumed inferior bone quality at the iliac crest. Finally, as with other bone-block procedures, this surgery is considered unsuitable for teenage patients with incomplete epiphyseal fusion at the iliac crest.

5.6 Surgical Technique

5.6.1 Preoperative Workup

While under endotracheal intubation and interscalene block, the patient is placed in the beach chair position and the ipsilateral iliac crest is exposed. Skin is disinfected from the forearm to the shoulder and over the hemithorax to the iliac crest, ending at the level of the greater trochanter. The arm is then draped loosely and rested on a table to the side.

5.6.2 Superficial Preparation

The landmarks for the skin incision are the tip of the coracoid process, the deltoid muscle and the axilla. The arm is held in a neutral position regarding flexion and extension in 30° of abduction and neutral rotation while it rests on the table. A skin incision of about 7 cm starting 1 cm lateral to the coracoid process and aiming toward the axilla is performed. After subcutaneous preparation and coagulation of small vessels, the deltopectoral interval is identified. Here, the cephalic vein lies between deltoid and pectoralis muscles. Along its medial aspect, the vein is now developed from proximal to distal by blunt preparation. In this procedure, the pectoralis muscle is separated from the deltoid muscle and the cephalic vein. Using a wide muscle retractor, the cephalic vein, along with the deltoid muscle, is retracted laterally; this is done because the cephalic vein is usually more adherent to the deltoid than to the pectoralis. Apart from this, a branch of the thoracoacromial artery lies parallel and lateral to this vein. This branch is then retracted and protected, along with the muscle that it partly supplies. The pectoralis muscle is retracted medially by a Langenbeck hook. Then, the subpectoral and subdeltoid spaces are developed by blunt preparation. The pectoral muscle is followed distally to its insertion at the humerus. Here, it is incised at a length of 5 mm for better exposure of the subscapularis tendon.

In the depth of the operation site, the short head of the biceps muscle is identified in the middle of the operating field. The muscle is followed cranially along with the coracobrachialis muscle, where they together insert as the conjoined tendon at the coracoid tip. Again, for better exposure of the subscapularis tendon at the lateral aspect of the coracoid tip, the conjoined tendon is horizontally incised at a length of 3 mm. Along the lateral aspect of the short biceps tendon, the soft tissue is separated by blunt preparation. The short biceps tendon is then retracted medially, along with the pectoralis major muscle, using the Langenbeck hook inserted previously. The mobilized deltoid muscle is now retracted laterally, and the subscapularis tendon is presented (Fig. 5.1).

Tips and Tricks

Often, the true deltopectoral interval lies more laterally than might be expected. Once the muscles are separated at the deltopectoral interval, further preparation can be done bluntly until the subscapularis tendon is developed. For better exposure of the subscapularis tendon, it is helpful but not essential to incise the pectoralis tendon at its insertion at the humerus and the conjoined tendon at the coracoid tip, as described.

Complications and Solutions

This step usually bears little risk for complications. When searching for the cephalic vein at the deltopectoral interval, it can be accidentally injured. In such cases, the vessel is ligated.

5.6.3 Subscapularis Incision

Adherent bursa tissue is removed from the subscapularis tendon. Again, by blunt preparation, the tendon is exposed for its entire extension from the lateral insertion at the lesser tuberosity medially to the muscle. Now, instead of detaching the tendon or performing an osteotomy of the lesser tuberosity, the tendon is split along its fibers where the middle and lower third meet (as seen from the frontal view). To prevent later bleeding from mucosal vessels, which are often relatively strong, the cautery is useful for the superficial incision (Fig. 5.2). After such superficial incisions, further preparation is

Fig. 5.1. Presentation of the subscapularis tendon

Fig. 5.2. Superficial incision of the subscapularis tendon

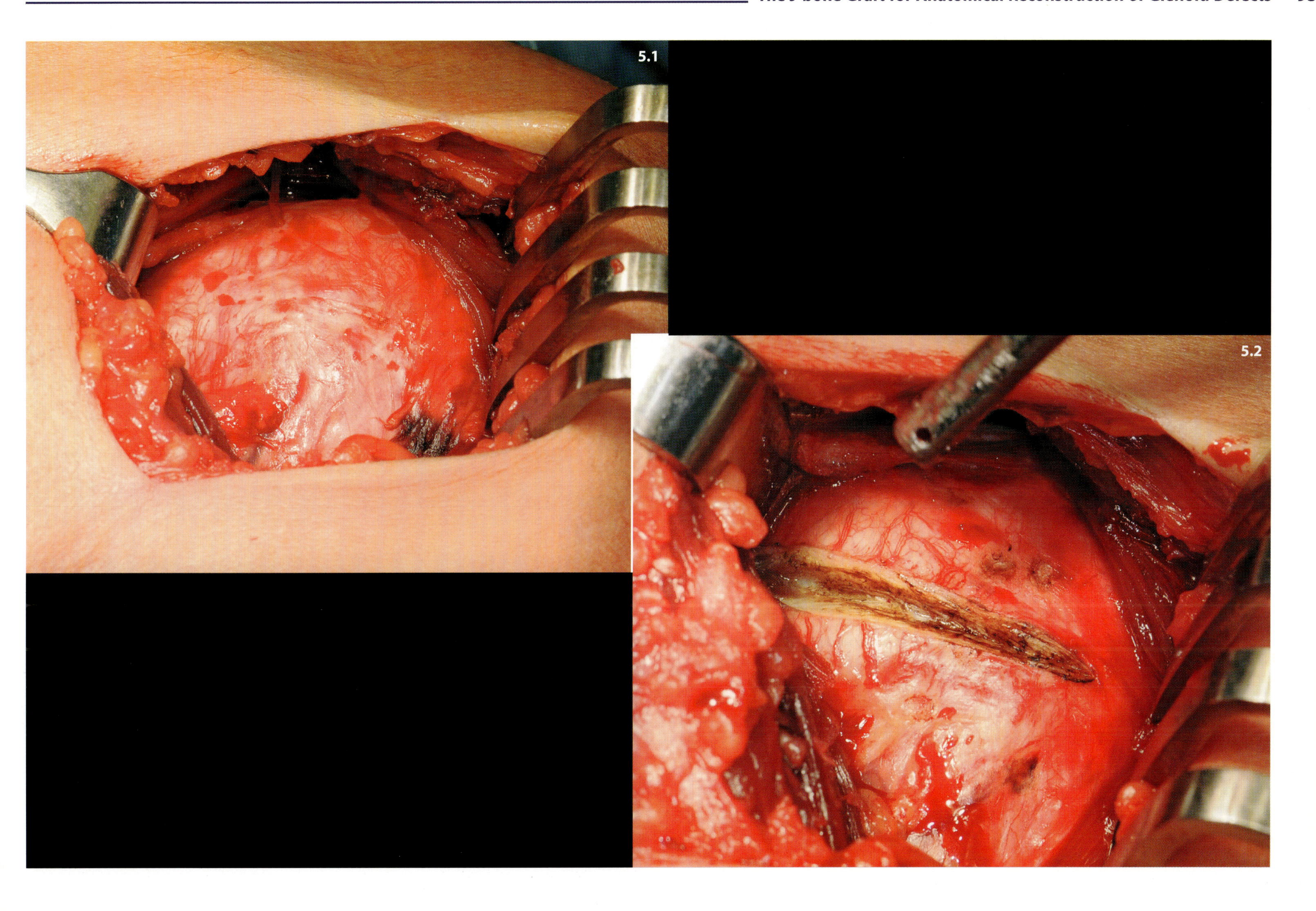
5.1
5.2

done using the scalpel (Fig. 5.3). The next step is to carefully separate the tendon from the underlying capsular tissue. At first, the tendon is split at a length of about 3 cm measured from the lesser tuberosity to the medial end of the incision. Once the capsule is identified, the tendon above it is retracted using a Gelpi retractor (MEDICON, D-78509 Tuttlingen, Germany). Separation of the tendon from the capsule in the medial direction is easiest and most safely accomplished using a rasp, which is inserted at the area where the tendon and capsule are already separated. When the medial end of the tendon-split is undermined with the rasp between the tendon and capsule, the rasp can then be slid down the capsule medially until the anteromedial glenoid is reached (Fig. 5.4). By flipping the rasp while it securely touches the bone, the medial aspect of the subscapularis tendon and the muscle are split along their fibers. With this blunt preparation for splitting the muscle, the axillary nerve, which runs over it, is secured.

Before splitting the capsule, the subscapularis tendon should be marked by one strong suture on the upper and lower sections where it is split. Next, the capsule is incised with the scalpel in line with the tendon split. When the capsule split has reached the glenoid rim, the rasp is positioned intra-articularly at the glenoid. Then, by blunt preparation further medially, a soft tissue sleeve of 1–1.5 cm consisting of periosteum and capsule is prepared with the

Fig. 5.3. Split of the subscapularis tendon

Fig. 5.4. Split of the subscapularis muscle

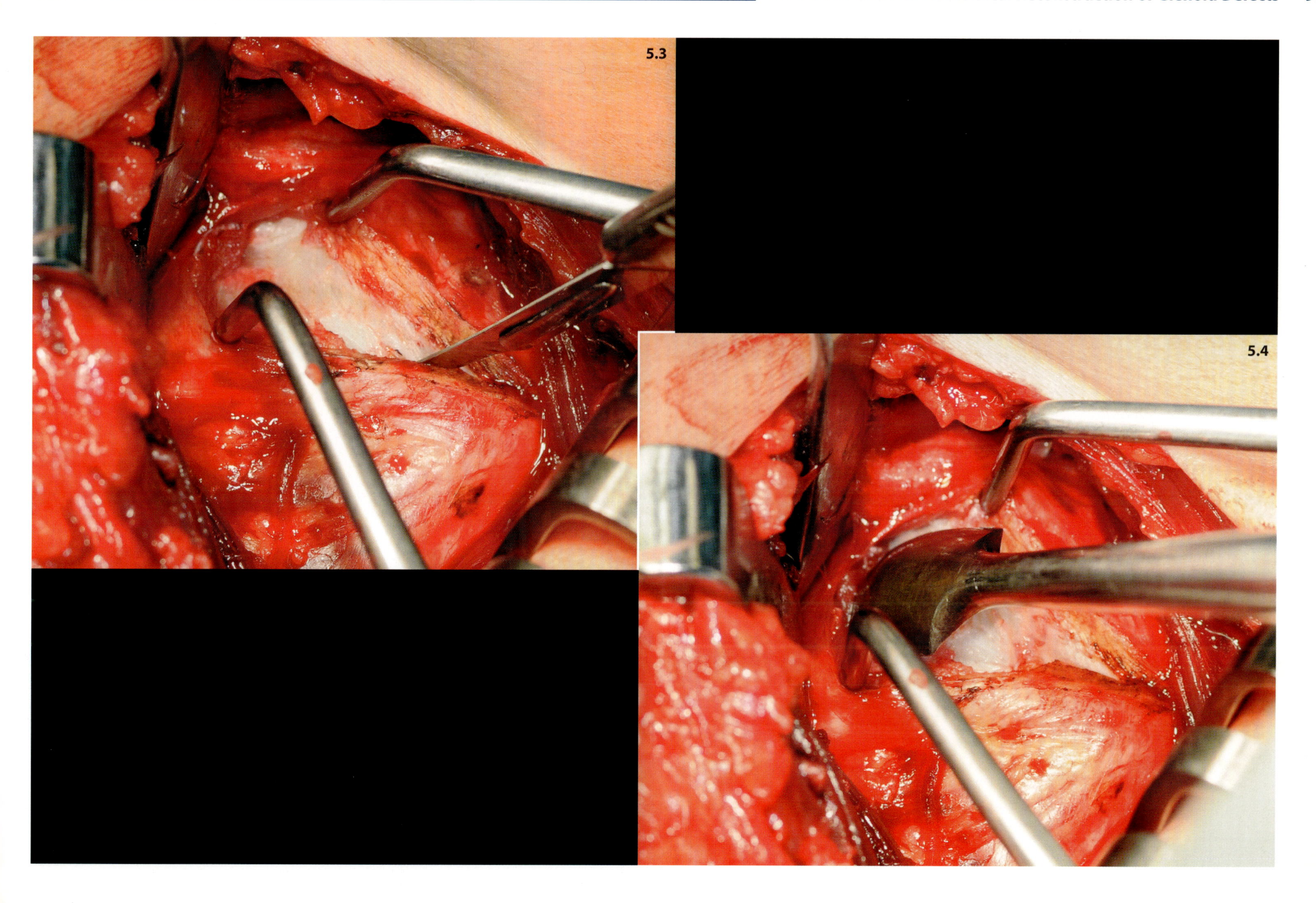
5.3
5.4

rasp. This sleeve is then incised. To later facilitate the suture of the capsule over the graft, the upper and lower rim of the split soft tissue should also be marked at this point by two strong sutures as medially as possible, because this part of the capsule will be hard to reach once the graft is in place (Fig. 5.5).

Tips and Tricks

The initial split of the subscapularis tendon must be performed accurately. To facilitate this, cauterization of the superficial vessels is helpful. Care must be taken to actually split the tendon along its fibers and not accidentally cut by an angled incision. The tendon can be 1- to 2-mm thick with a dorsally adherent capsule, so the incision with the scalpel should be performed with caution to prevent cutting through the tendon and capsule at the same time.

Complications and Solutions

If the capsule is accidentally incised along with the tendon, both layers can usually still be separated at the incision. When the layers are identified, further preparation can be continued as described above. If the capsule cannot be identified as a separate layer, which can occur in cases of revision surgery, the subscapularis tendon is split along with the adherent capsule. In such cases, the later suture of the tendon must start as medially as possible to enclose the graft for intra-articular positioning.

5.6.4 Glenoid Presentation

Once the subscapularis tendon and capsule are accurately split and the medial sutures are set in place, the rasp is exchanged for a spiked Hohmann retractor, which is positioned intra-articularly and medially at the scapular neck. This presents the glenoid rim defect. To now fully expose the glenoid rim, the humeral head is retracted by a Fukuda retractor (Smith & Nephew, London, UK). A second Hohmann retractor is then placed at the glenoid neck so that one sits at 6 o'clock and the other at 9 o'clock. The extent of the defect can now be accurately inspected. Larger or smaller fragments of former Bankart lesions can sometimes be identified at this point. Such fragments can more or less adhere to the glenoid rim or scapular neck, but they usually lie in an extra-anatomic position. These findings will not be surprising, however, because preoperative imaging always reveals such situations. Intraoperatively, such fragments are practically always embedded in a soft tissue layer, which partly consists of the former labrum. In situ, they can appear to be more or less resorbed or, less often, may be covered by cartilage-like tissue. As the next step, the former labrum is incised in line with the incision of the capsule, and the osseous fragment is peeled out of the soft tissue surrounding it and is removed. Then, the usually intact parts of the labrum cranial and caudal to the defect site are mobilized with the rasp. In this procedure, the glenoid rim defect must

Fig. 5.5. Positioning the medial capsular sutures

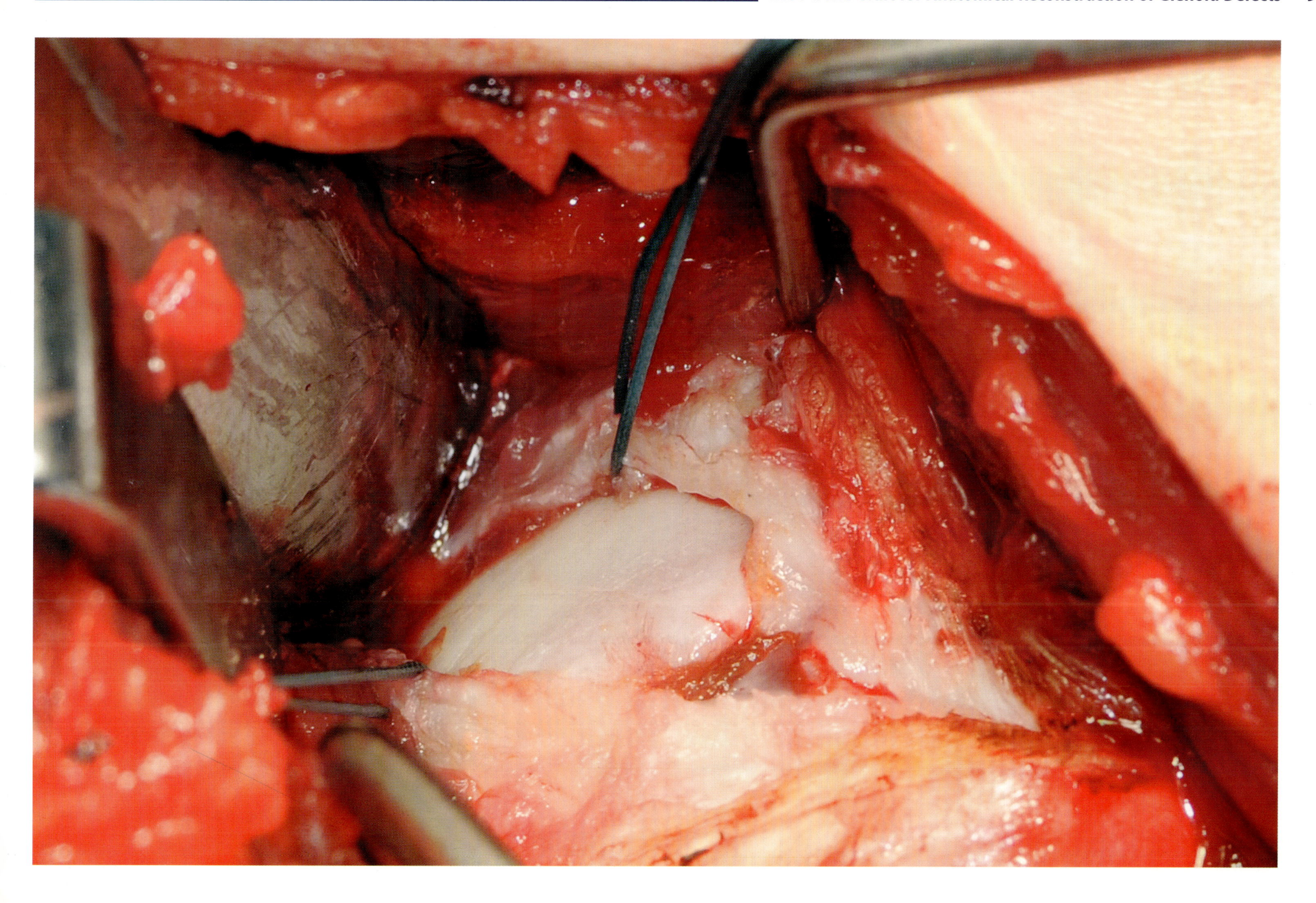

be presented to see its full dimension (Fig. 5.6). Finally, the defect site at the glenoid rim is cleaned of any adherent soft tissue and carefully prepared with a rasp to leave a triangular plane of slightly bleeding spongy bone. The wound is now tamponaded with a wet swab, and the surgeon proceeds to harvest the bone graft from the ipsilateral iliac crest.

Tips and Tricks

For easy positioning of the retractor used for the humeral head, the shoulder should be held in slight internal rotation. When inspecting the glenoid rim, the labrum can always be identified. Usually, it is partly degenerated and lies further medially than it would when uninjured. In most cases, the labrum is reduced in size and runs directly over the defect site. If there is still an adherent osseous fragment at the glenoid, it usually is adherent to this former rim. Only in very few cases will such a fragment appear to be of substantially better quality than would have been suspected on preoperative images. If this is the case, as a change in procedure, the fragment could be fixed to the glenoid rim after preparation of the defect site, as described above. This is done with two cannulated 2.7-mm screws, as in acute glenoid-rim fractures. When the degenerated labrum goes around an osseous fragment that needs to be removed, it may be wide enough to later suture it over the graft before suturing the capsule. In such a case, after incising the labrum as described above, both ends should be armed with strong sutures to later achieve closure over the graft. If the labrum cannot be closed over the graft, the sutures should be removed.

Complications and Solutions

Careless medial placement of the Hohmann retractor at the glenoid neck can cause damage to the brachial plexus. To avoid this, it is necessary to always keep it on the bone during preparation of the glenoid neck. Preparation must be done stepwise and carefully. Positioning the spiked Hohmann retractor about 2 cm medial of the cartilage surface provides enough space for further preparation. If a former osseous fragment has healed to the glenoid further medially, it can be left in place when it sits at least 1 cm medial to the cartilage surface. Any bone or soft tissue lateral to that point must be completely removed to avoid later constraint of the graft fixation.

Fig. 5.6. Presentation of the glenoid defect

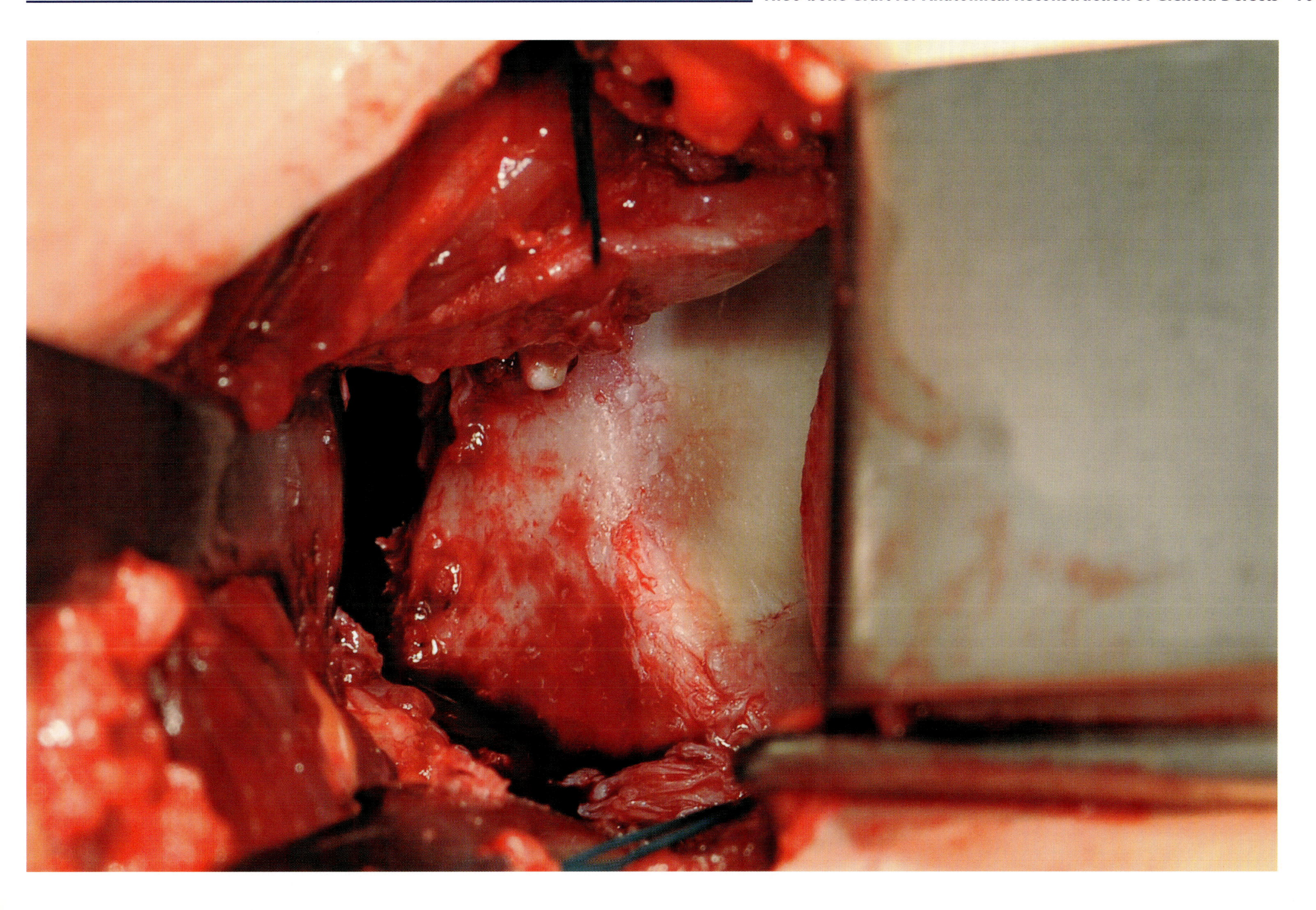

5.6.5 Harvesting the Graft

A skin incision 5 cm long starting 5 cm posterior to the ipsilateral superior iliac spine over the iliac crest is made. To expose the crest, subcutaneous fat is split with the cautery to reach the periosteum of the iliac crest. The periosteum is then incised with the cautery or the scalpel, as preferred. Using a rasp or elevator, the medial and lateral portion of the periosteal sleeve is mobilized and then retracted, along with the muscle tissue, using a spiked Hohmann retractor. With the iliac crest now fully exposed, the width of the blank graft is marked with the cautery. The J-bone graft is a bicortical iliac crest graft, which when prepared should be 15 mm wide, 5 mm high, and 15 mm long with a triangular shape. To avoid taking a graft that is too slim, a distance of 18 mm is marked. Using the oscillating saw, a cut of about 2 cm deep involving all three cortices is performed. The height of each individual blank graft depends on the width of the iliac crest. Next, the inner cortex is left in place. Using the oscillating saw, an incision is made starting medially at the upper cortex aiming laterally at the outer cortex to the point where the first two incisions ended (Fig. 5.7). Depending on the blade used, this incision usually ends just behind the outer cortex, which is then cut through with a chisel. Now, a wedge-shaped bone block of 15- to 18-mm wide, 5- to 10-mm high, and approximately 20-mm long is created (Fig. 5.8) The donor site is covered with a hemostatic sponge, and the wound is closed in layers.

Tips and Tricks

A shorter skin incision and subcutaneous preparation with the diathermy at the iliac crest can reduce donor-site morbidity. Theoretically, the width of the graft can be varied depending on the width of the actual glenoid defect. In our experience, however, a width of 15 mm fits practically all cases. The blank bone block can be taken a few millimeters wider to avoid a graft that is too narrow. The third incision with the oscillating saw need not run exactly from the upper inner cortex to the lower outer cortex. The objective is not to harvest the graft in just three steps but to spare the inner cortex from damage, as it often is convex to the outer side.

Complications and Solutions

This step usually bears little risk of complications. Marks for the incisions should indicate a graft slightly larger than finally needed. If the inner cortex of the iliac crest is cut by the last incision, a tricortical bone block may result. This can make further graft modeling slightly more complex but has no other side effects. Special care should be taken, however, not to accidentally cut the outer cortex by holding the saw at an overly inclined angle. This could leave a keel too short for secure graft fixation. In such a case, the graft might need to be additionally secured by one cannulated 2.7-mm titanium screw for reliable anchorage.

Fig. 5.7. Harvest of the bone block

Fig. 5.8. Appearance of the bone block before shaping the J-bone graft

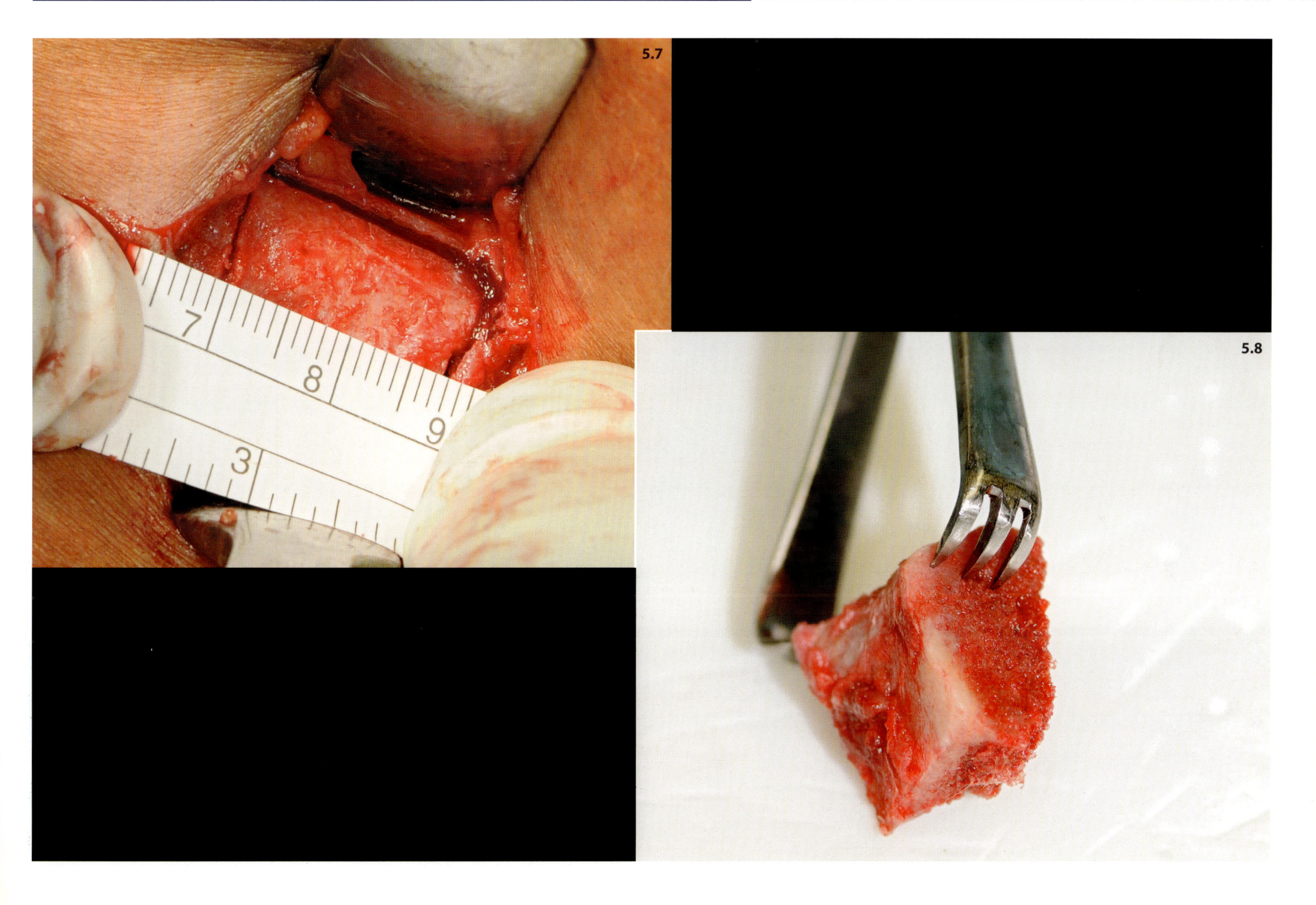
5.7
7
8
9
3
5.8

5.6.6 J-bone-graft Modelling

For this step, the surgeon must take time to carefully model the graft out of the harvested bone block. The blank graft is now held with a spiked forceps to ensure it does not slip away during modeling. At this point, it can be narrowed to 15 mm if it was originally wider. For the part of the graft that is meant to restore the missing glenoid rim, a block 5 mm wide consisting of the upper cortex and cancellous bone is left. The remaining cancellous bone is removed from the outer cortex, which will form the cortical keel. For these two incisions, the oscillating saw is used (Figs. 5.9 and 5.10). Next, the remaining cancellous bone is cleared from the keel; this can also

Fig. 5.9. Vertical incision to separate cancellous bone from the graft's keel

Fig. 5.10. Horizontal incision to separate cancellous bone from the graft's keel

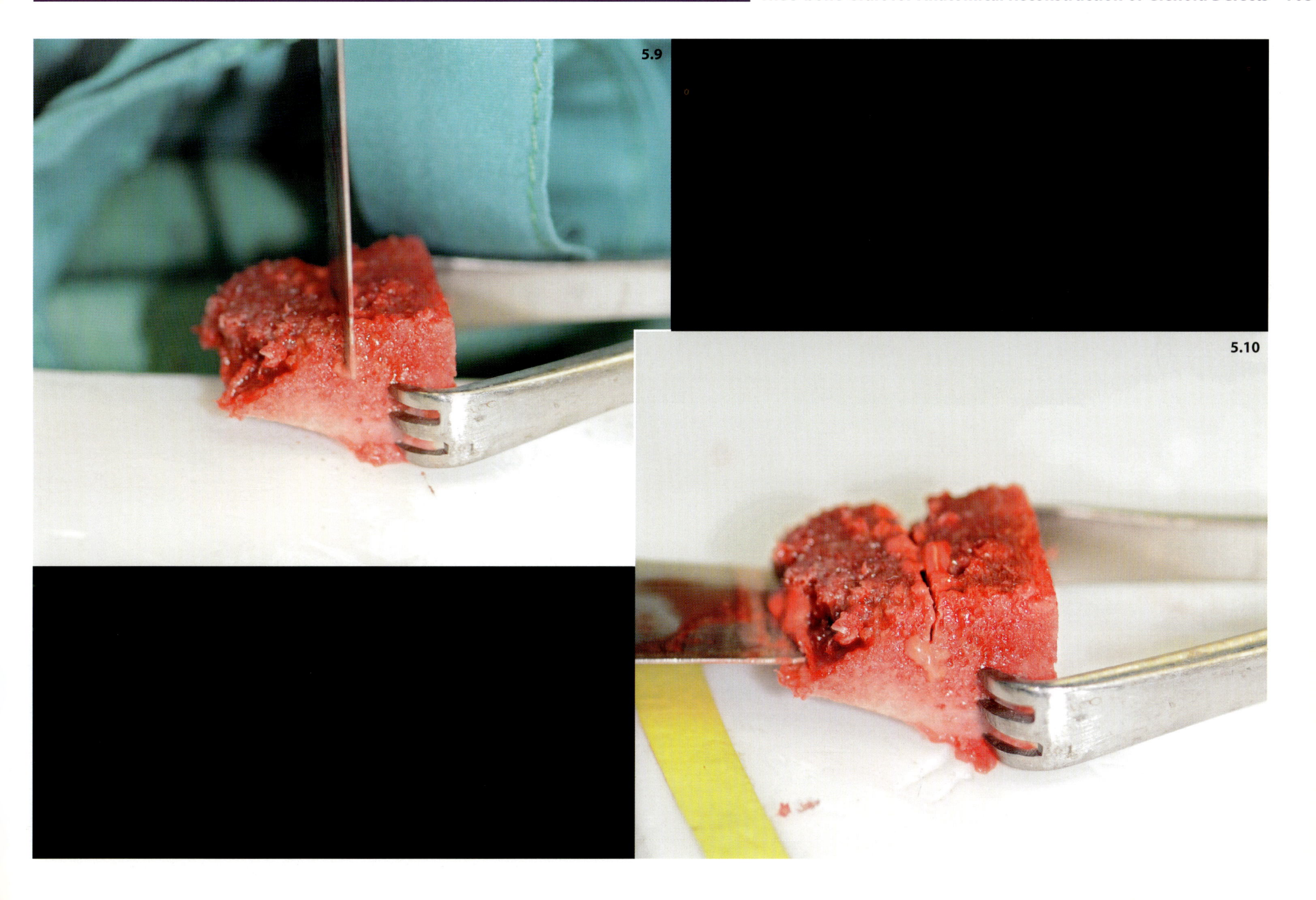
5.9
5.10

be done with the saw, or alternatively, with a high-speed burr (Fig. 5.11). Next, the keel is shortened to 10 mm, the edges are trimmed, and it is thinned at the end so it can later slip unimpeded into its preformed crevice. Finally, in profile, the modeled graft looks like the letter J (Fig. 5.12).

Tips and Tricks

During preparation, it is essential to securely hold the graft with the spiked forceps, as it can easily fall. For this purpose, we recommend using a cutting board placed on an extra table on which the surgeon's forearms can rest to facilitate secure instrumentation. Care should be taken not to thin out the entire keel. Only the tip is trimmed; for the rest of the keel, only cancellous bone is removed. At this point, the height of the graft has not yet been corrected. This will only be done when the graft is securely positioned.

Complications and Solutions

The first possible complication during this step is that the graft can fall during preparation. If this happens, a second graft must be harvested from the iliac crest. Embedding the graft in antiseptic solution for a few minutes is not recommended. When removing the spare cancellous bone, the vertical incision, in particular, must be carefully made so as not to cut through the cortex of the keel. If that occurs, the advantage of stable screwless fixation is lost. When a true J-bone-graft procedure is performed, a second graft is harvested. Alternatively, the graft can be fixed by two cannulated 2.7-mm titanium screws. When positioning such screws, their heads must lie at least 3 mm below the glenoid surface to make sure they do not touch the humeral head. Rates of graft nonunion or resorption are not known for such cases. If by the horizontal incision the graft's keel is weakened by mistake, the stability of its integration has to be tested in situ. Because the thickness of each patient's cortex at the iliac crest is different, this may not cause a problem in all cases.

Fig. 5.11. Shaping the graft's kee

Fig. 5.12. Preshaped J-bone graft

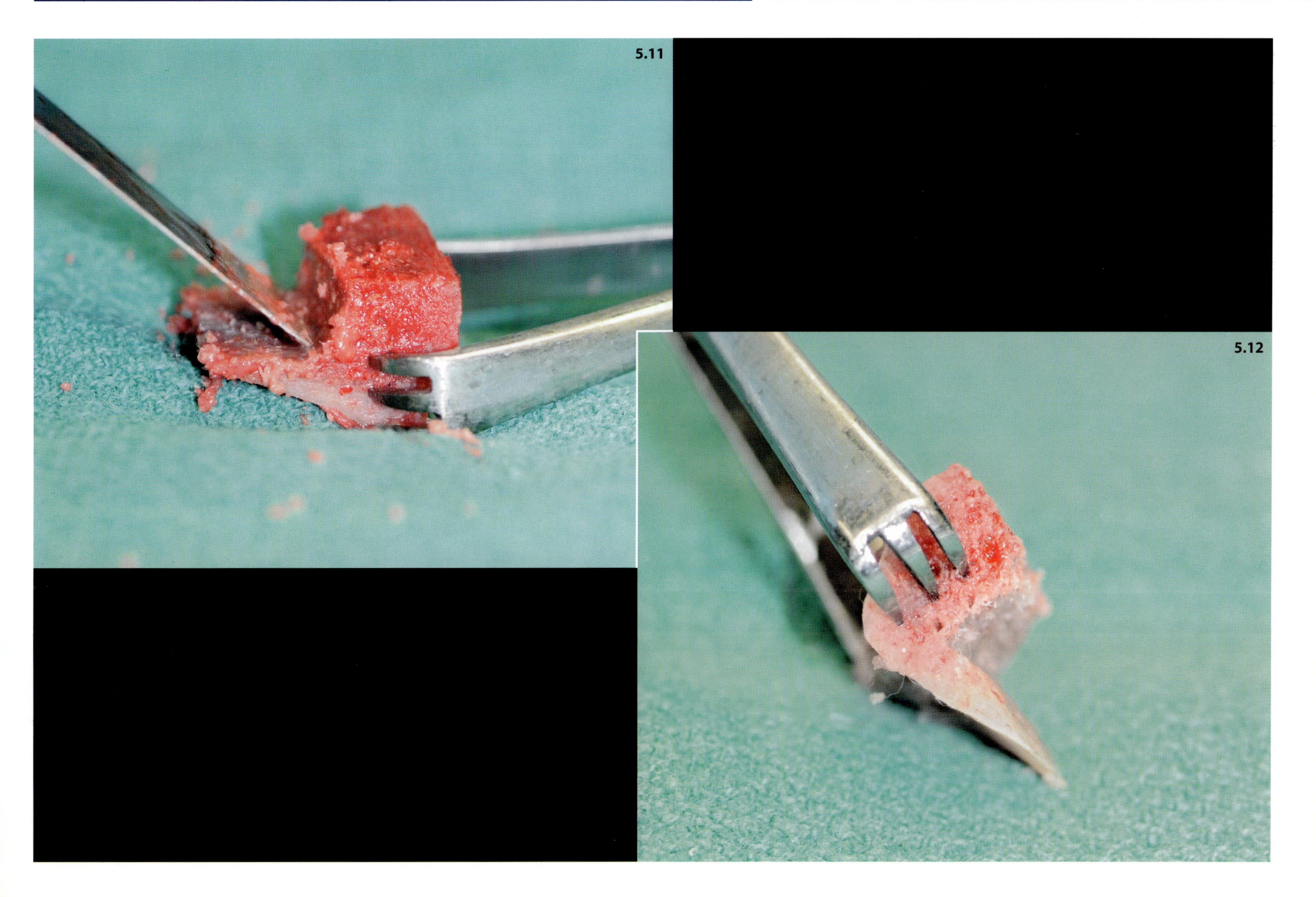
5.11
5.12

5.6.7 Glenoid Osteotomy

To hold the graft without screw fixation, an osteotomy at the glenoid neck must be performed. Apart from modeling the graft, this step often is assumed to be the most delicate. Surgeons inexperienced with the procedure usually fear causing a glenoid-neck fracture when doing this osteotomy. We have never seen this complication; it can easily be avoided by keeping in mind the following instructions. To perform the osteotomy, a common chisel 10-mm wide and 15-mm long is used. As with all chisels, the instrument is thinner at the tip and thicker at its base. The tamponade is removed from the operation site. The soft tissue is retracted using the hooks at 9 and 6 o'clock, and the wound is rinsed. The osteotomy is initiated in the middle of the defect site. The chisel must now be placed 5 mm medial to the cartilage surface of the intact glenoid with the blade parallel to the rim of the defect. Before starting with the osteotomy, the instrument must be additionally inclined at 30°, aiming medially (Fig. 5.13). This position is maintained until the blade

Fig. 5.13. Positioning the chisel for the osteotomy at the glenoid neck

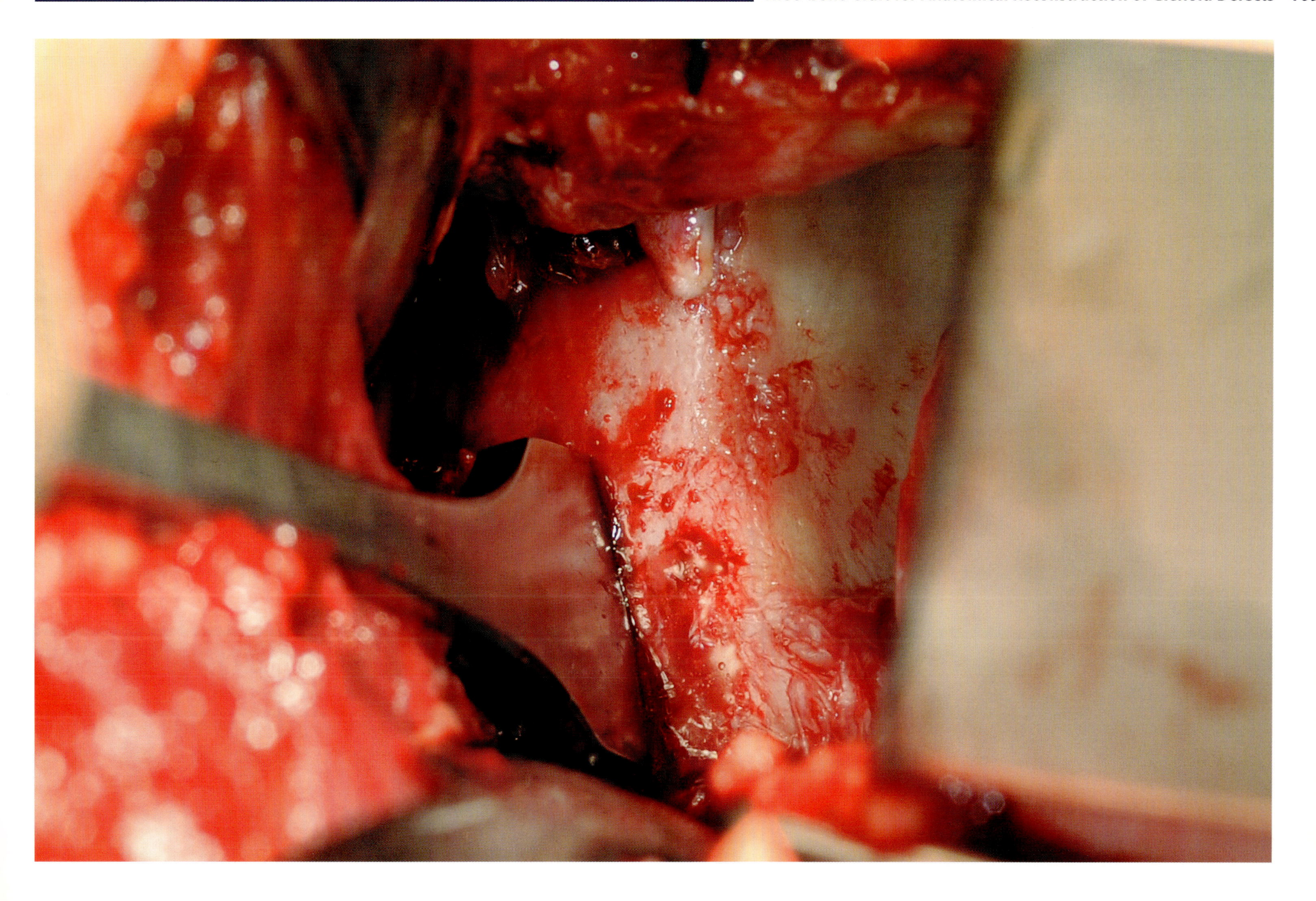

is sunk into the shoulder, which will produce a crevice 15-mm deep. This procedure is now repeated to continually elongate the osteotomy from its center to the upper and lower edges (Fig. 5.14). In the end, a crevice 25-mm long, 2-mm wide, and – depending on the chisel used – about 15-mm deep is prepared.

Tips and Tricks

This is the step with which most surgeons initially feel uncomfortable. It is necessary to place the chisel and incline it as described. If the plane of the intact glenoid fossa is not easy to assess, a rasp can be laid on it upside down to indicate its inclination. A safe grip is necessary to prevent slippage off the defect site further medially. When the first crevice is produced, it should be lengthened stepwise in a vertical direction, keeping the crevice parallel to the glenoid rim. For this purpose, the instrument should partly rest in the preformed crevice instead of producing a second one next to it. This ensures that the plane of the preformed slot is maintained. Each time the chisel is newly positioned during this procedure, it must be carefully loosened because it usually gets stuck in the tight crevice produced. When repositioning the instrument, caution must be taken to not bend it horizontally, as this could lever the articular surface. Rather, it must be moved vertically.

Complications and Solutions

In case a glenoid-neck fracture occurs, the chipped-off fragment must be reduced and fixed by one or two cannulated 2.7-mm titanium screws, and the procedure must be aborted. The wound is closed as described below. After about 2 months, when the fragment should be fully healed, a second attempt could be made. The crevice should not lie further medial than 5 mm below the cartilage surface, because at this point, the axial diameter of the glenoid neck is the widest. If it does, this does not necessarily cause a problem as long as no glenoid-neck fracture results. Depending on the width of the patient's iliac crest, the initial height of the graft can vary. When the crevice is correctly positioned, it is usually necessary to reduce this height by a few millimeters. In this respect, further medialization of the crevice can be compensated. This is also the reason that the graft height is adjusted in situ. If the chisel is moved horizontally when being loosened, the crevice can be widened by mistake. If this results in weak graft fixation, one cannulated 2.7-mm titanium screw must be inserted to secure the graft.

Fig. 5.14. Completed osteotomy at the glenoid neck

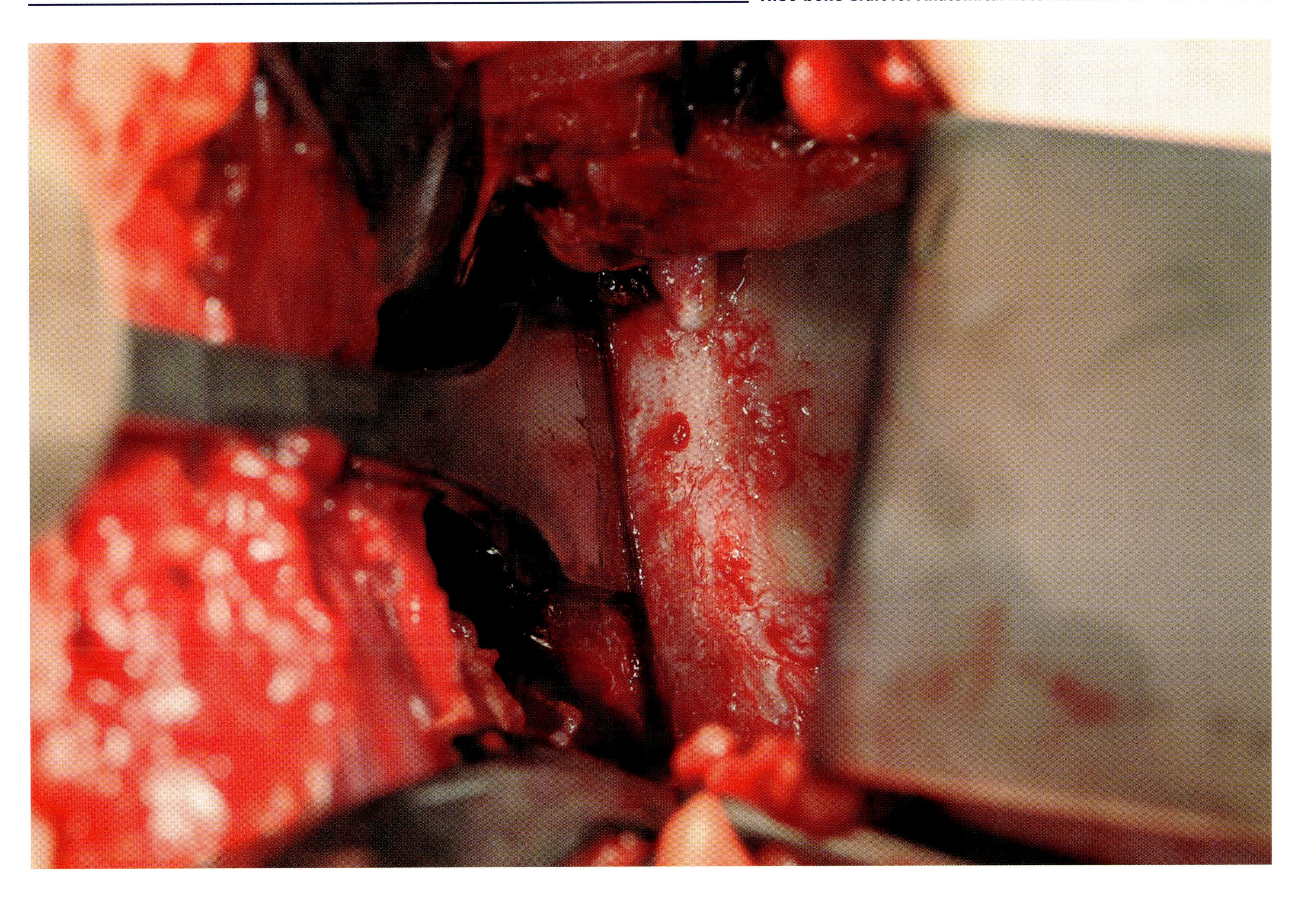

5.6.8 Graft Positioning

Holding the J-bone graft with the spiked forceps, the graft's keel of cancellous bone is now fitted in the preformed crevice. Before using an impactor and hammer to fit the graft tight, it must be correctly positioned by hand. While the graft is held with a forceps, it can be tilted back and forth vertically until it seems to fit tightly. During this process, its position should be controlled, making sure it sits in the center of the defect. Then, to ensure axial stress only and to prevent the graft from slipping off, a spiked impactor (Synthes, Solothurn, Switzerland) is placed at the rim of the graft where the upper cortex merges to the lateral cortex of the former iliac crest (Fig. 5.15) As with the chisel earlier in the procedure, this impactor must be held at 30° of inclination. When a secure grip is ensured,

Fig. 5.15. Fitting the graft into the produced crevice using the spiked impactor

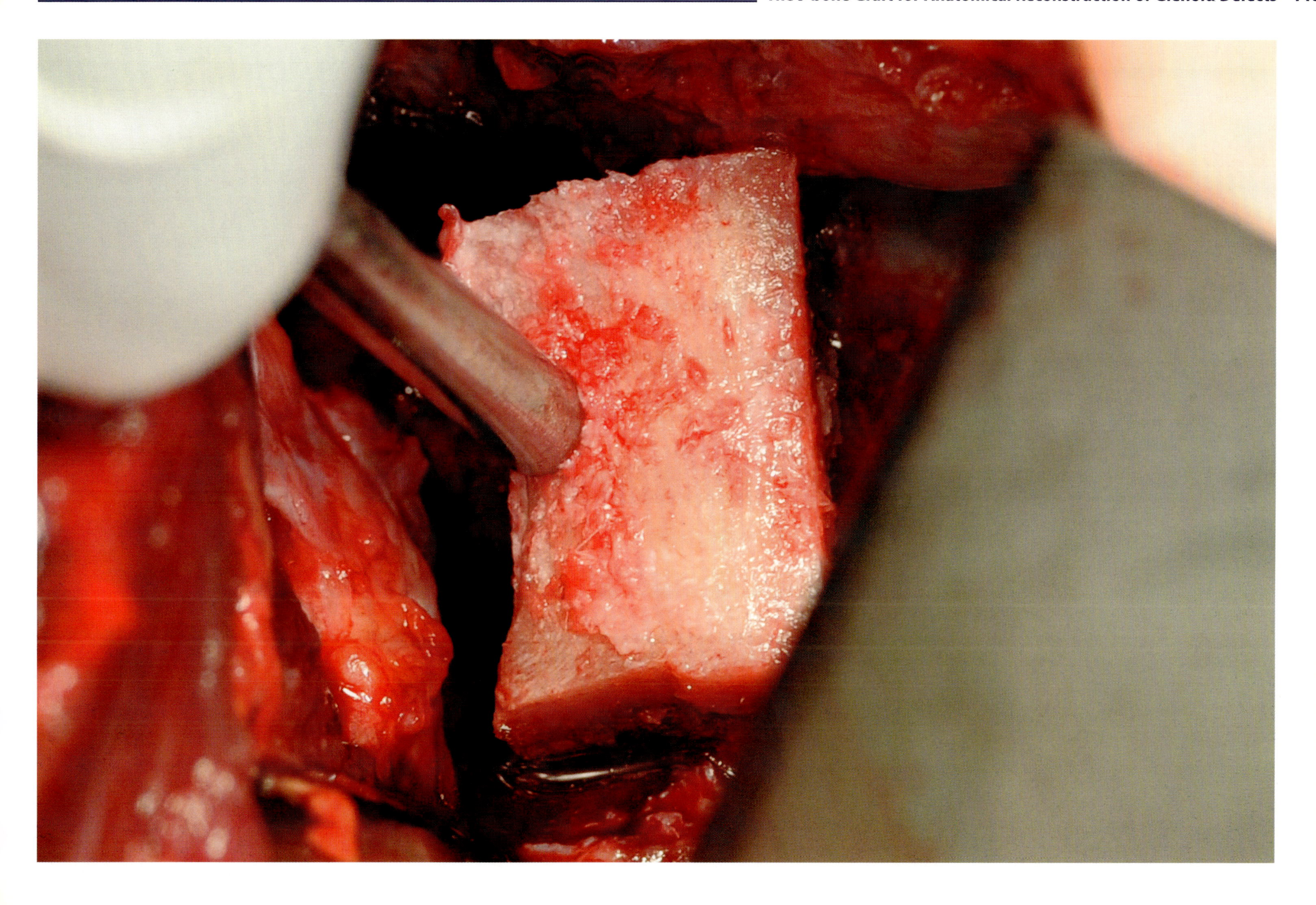

the graft is hammered further in. The body of the graft is then tightly impacted into the former glenoid defect site, leaving no gap. When the graft is in place, its surface is trimmed to restore the former cavity of the glenoid using an olive-shaped burr (Fig. 5.16). This should produce a seamless transition between cartilage and the graft's cancellous bone (Fig. 5.17).

Tips and Tricks

When inserting the graft by hand, it is important not to bend the keel horizontally but to only tilt the graft vertically in the plane of the keel to prevent a fracture. As mentioned above, the thickness of the patient's cortical bone can vary; therefore, the keel can be more or less fragile. When it is impacted and has full contact with the former defect but still seems to be resilient, it can be secured by one cannulated 2.7-mm titanium screw. This screw should be positioned 3 mm below the articular surface inclined at 20°. Recent investigations show that the graft will soon be covered by cartilage-like tissue. Because this layer of cartilage may then overlap with the rest of the articular cartilage, trimming the graft 1 mm below the cartilage surface has been discussed as an option.

Complications and Solutions

Once the graft is readily impacted, its position is difficult to correct without damaging it. If correction is nonetheless necessary, again, the graft must be tilted only in the plane of the keel. If the graft's keel fractures during impaction or when trying to correct its position, as described above, it should be screwed to the glenoid.

5.6.9 Closing the Wound

When enclosing the bone graft, the arm should be held in 60° abduction and 30° external rotation. In case the humeral head gains contact with the graft in this position, the graft must be shaped with the burr to avoid such contact. In case the labrum is wide enough, the surgeon can attempt to suture it over the graft using the sutures set in place earlier. If this does not work because the labrum has shrunk and degenerated, it should simply be left in place. The joint capsule, which was previously marked by two strong sutures, can always be sutured over the graft, fully enclosing it for intra-articular positioning. In the same way, the split of the subscapularis tendon is closed by strong nonabsorbable sutures. The muscle retractors are removed so the pectoralis and deltoid muscles again lie side by side without sutures. A wound drain is positioned, the subcutaneous layer is sutured by absorbable material, and the skin is stapled.

Tips and Tricks

To prevent postoperative arthropathy, the point at which graft and humeral head touch each other must be identified. The surgeon himself holds the arm in position to test this interference. In cases of doubt, the graft should be thinned out slightly rather than risking humeral-head loading. It can be a rather time consuming attempt trying to suture the capsule over the graft without previously having positioned the medial sutures, so positioning these sutures right after splitting the capsule is strongly recommended. With these sutures in place, it is easy to close the capsule over the relatively prominent bone block.

Fig. 5.16. Shaping the graft's surface in situ

Fig. 5.17. Final appearance of the J-bone graft before wound closure

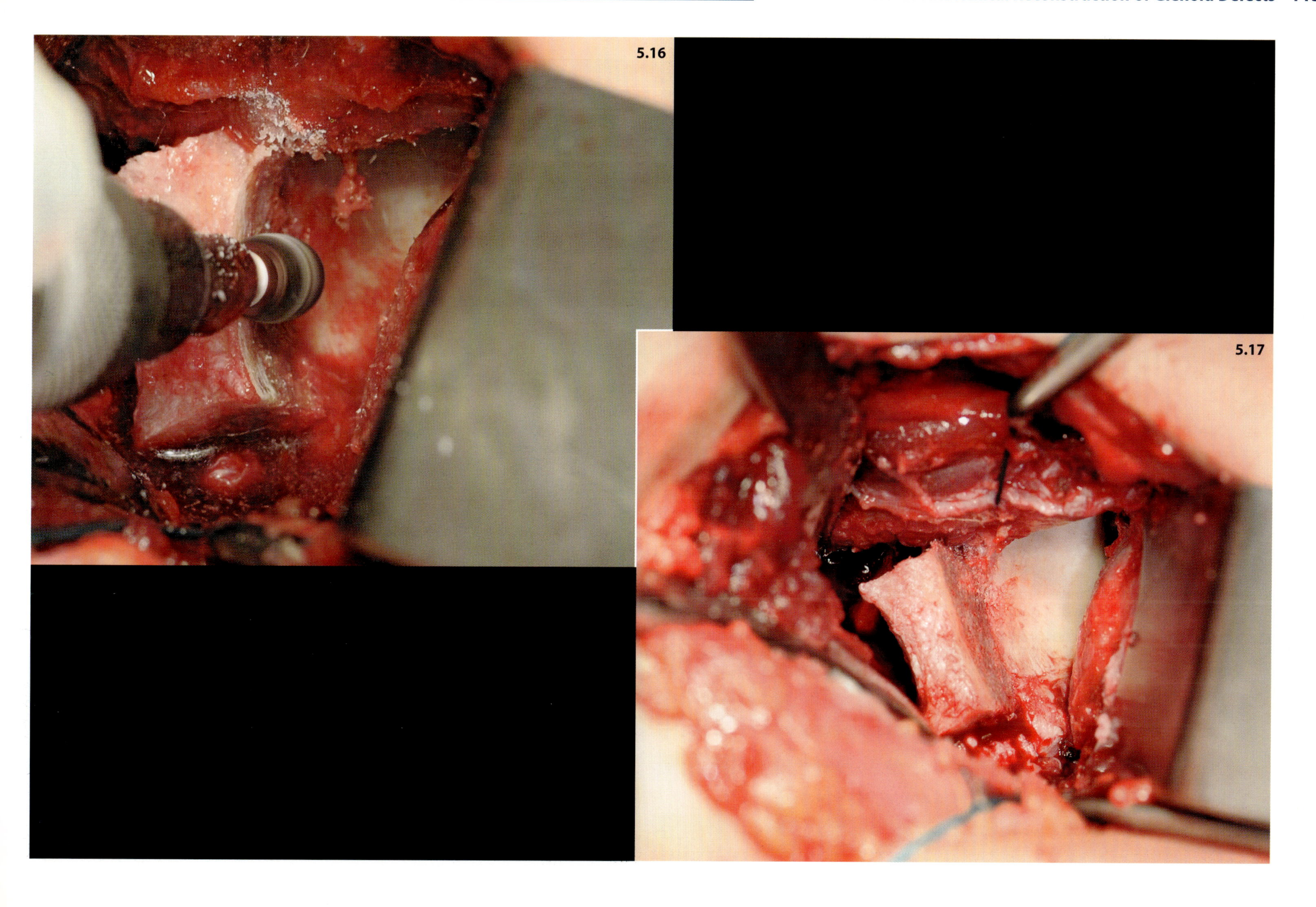
5.16
5.17

Complications and Solutions

Closing the wound is rather uncomplicated as long as the sutures described above were positioned correctly.

5.7 Postoperative Care

Postoperative Weeks 1–4

- sling for 3 weeks;
- finger and elbow gymnastics are allowed;
- pendular exercises;
- isometric exercises;
- sling must be worn except during showering and passive physical therapy.

Postoperative Weeks 5 and 6

- sling is removed;
- passive and active motion is allowed to the following extent:
  - flexion 90°
  - extension 30°
  - abduction 30°
- external rotation to neutral position;
- internal rotation to the onset of pain.

Postoperative Weeks 7–12

- active motion allowed to the onset of pain, and exercises should be intensified step by step;
- muscular strengthening.

After 12 Weeks

- all sports, except for throwing and overhead sports, are allowed.

After 16 Weeks

- sports are allowed with no restriction.

Complementary Measures

- cryotherapy;
- lymph drainage;
- electrical stimulation:
  - for analgesic use starting the first postoperative week;
  - for muscular stimulation starting the fifth postoperative week;
  - underwater therapy starting the fifth postoperative week.

References

1. Gerber C, Nyffeler RW (2002) Classification of glenohumeral joint instability. Clin Orthop Relat Res 400:65-76
2. Sugaya H, Moriishi J, Kanisawa I, Tsuchiya A (2005) Arthroscopic osseous Bankart repair for chronic recurrent traumatic anterior glenohumeral instability. J Bone Joint Surg Am 87:1752-1760
3. Bigliani LU, Newton PM, Steinmann SP et al (1998) Glenoid rim lesions associated with recurrent anterior dislocation of the shoulder. Am J Sports Med 26:41-45
4. Itoi E, Lee SB, Berglund L et al (2000) The effect of a glenoid defect on anteroinferior stability of the shoulder after Bankart repair: a cadaveric study. J Bone Joint Surg Am 82:35-46
5. Montgomery WH, Wahl M, Hettrich C et al (2005) Anteroinferior bone-grafting can restore stability in osseous glenoid defects. J Bone Joint Surg Am 87:1972-1977
6. Kartus C, Kartus J, Matis N et al (2008) Long-term independent evaluation after arthroscopic extra-articular Bankart repair with absorbable tacks. Surgical technique. J Bone Joint Surg Am 90(Suppl 2 Pt 2):262-274
7. Auffarth A, Schauer J, Matis N et al (2008) The J-bone graft for anatomical glenoid reconstruction in recurrent posttraumatic anterior shoulder dislocation. Am J Sports Med 36:638-647
8. Tauber M, Resch H, Forstner R et al (2004) Reasons for failure after surgical repair of anterior shoulder instability. J Shoulder Elbow Surg 13:279-285

Chapter 6 – Iliac-crest Graft and Distal Tibia Allograft Procedure

Matthew T. Provencher, Andrew R. Hsu, Neil S. Ghodadra and Anthony A. Romeo

6.1 Introduction

Glenohumeral stability depends on active and passive restraints as well as coordinated interactions between the rotator-cuff muscles and bony structures to properly maintain the humeral head within the glenoid. Glenohumeral instability is a pathologic state in which excessive translation of the humeral head within the glenoid leads to pain, decreased range of motion, impaired functional status, and subluxation or dislocation. This may be a result of injury to the labrum, capsule, ligaments, rotator-cuff muscles, or bony articular surface. The labrum is an important structure that deepens the glenoid fossa and serves as a static stabilizer and attachment for capsuloligamentous structures, and the glenoid is a critical structure that helps maintain static restraint of the humerus [1]. Traumatic bony insults causing glenoid-bone deficiency are a common reason for recurrent anterior shoulder instability and capsulolabral reconstruction failure. Glenoid reconstruction can be surgically challenging, and there are a number of reconstruction techniques, including coracoid transfer [2, 3], iliac-crest autograft [4, 5], allograft glenoid tissue, and other allograft tissue, such as the femoral head, and osteochondral allografts such as the distal tibia [6].

6.2 History

Clinical history of shoulder instability is a key element of whether or not to pursue surgical intervention for glenoid lesions, as several factors have been found to affect instability recurrence, including patient age and involvement in contact sports and shoulder hyperlaxity. It is necessary to assess the presence of an initial traumatic event as well as mechanism of injury to determine the likelihood of concurrent injuries such as glenoid fractures, capsular and rotator-cuff tears, and capsulolabral disruption [7]. Glenoid lesions are found in 22% of patients with acute dislocations and 73% with recurrent dislocations [8]. Therefore, it is important to determine onset, chronology, and frequency of dislocation events as well as any acute nonsurgical or surgical interventions. It is also vital to rule out voluntary dislocation as a possible cause of instability. Attention should be paid to symptoms such as pain, weakness, paresthesias, popping, clicking, and instability during range of motion and activities of daily living. Patient baseline functional status, participation in sports or high levels of physical activity, level of disability, and subjective reports such as arm positions and activities avoided due to pain are key indicators of the level of glenohumeral instability and laxity. It is essential to assess patient expectations and desires for functional status after potential surgery to match surgical outcomes as best as possible with benefits from procedures.

6.3 Examination

Physical examination is an important aspect of the workup of shoulder instability and can provide important clues for patients with symptomatic bone loss. The examination should begin with inspection of the shoulder contour, muscle symmetry, and passive and active range of motion. The exam should then focus on generalized ligamentous laxity, global laxity (anterior, posterior, inferior), and potential subluxation and dislocation of the glenohumeral joint [9]. Generalized laxity should be assessed to include hyperextension of the thumbs and elbows and genu recurvatum. Patient arm position at baseline should be noted for exaggerated internal or external rotation and the presence of a prominent anterior or posterior shoulder, giving clues as to the direction of instability. Anteroposterior translation of the humerus can be assessed using the load-and-shift test, with grade 1 having increased translation but no subluxation, grade 2 with humeral-head subluxation over the glenoid with spontaneous reduction, and grade 3 having humeral-head dislocation over the glenoid rim. The load-and-shift test will identify the direction of instability and must be performed in the plane of the scapula with the scapula stabilized.

Physical examination may also provide important clues to the presence of glenoid or humeral-head bone loss. Decreased resistance to anterior shift, along with possible crepitus or grinding, will be felt with an anterior glenoid-rim lesion. Patients with apprehension and guarding at lower degrees of abduction and external rotation are more likely to have larger anterior bony glenoid lesions. In addition, apprehension at midabduction and midexternal rotation is highly suggestive of the presence of glenoid-bone loss.

Tips and Tricks

- In patients who describe instability in midranges of motion, carefully assess for glenoid-bone loss;
- in patients who demonstrate instability with the arm abducted <45°, carefully screen for glenoid-bone loss.

6.4 Imaging

Radiographs for evaluating potential glenoid-bone loss should include a shoulder anteroposterior X-ray done 30° to the shoulder-joint surface, a scapular X-ray, and an axillary view of the affected shoulder [8]. The transthoracic or outlet X-ray can be helpful in determining the direction of dislocation. With suspected glenoid-bone loss, it is helpful to use the West Point view and for Hill-Sachs lesions the Stryker notch view. Itoi et al. have shown that the West Point view has a high correlation with computed tomography (CT) in estimating glenoid-bone loss [10]. Glenoid-bone loss from recurrent instability and bone resorption leads to an inverted pear-shaped glenoid that is wider superiorly than it is inferiorly. There is a strong association between the severity of the bony glenoid defects and the incidence of recurrent instability. The length of the glenoid defect is measured along the anterior edge, with attention being paid to the length relative to the maximum anteroposterior diameter of the glenoid fossa. If there is significant anterior glenoid erosion, the superoinferior axis of the glenoid can be measured with respect to the radius of the glenoid fossa [5, 11].

CT scan of the humeral head with 3D reconstruction and digital subtraction is useful for more detailed evaluation of bony anatomy for preoperative evaluation of glenoid-bone loss [12]. CT is indicated when the patient has significant apprehension during physical exam and multiple instability events and if any bone loss is seen on X-ray. Previous studies have found that CT arthrogram with gadolinium also accurately reflects bony glenoid lesions [5, 11]. Magnetic resonance imaging (MRI) can be added to visualize concomitant pathology, including soft-tissue injuries, labral lesions, humeral avulsion of the glenohumeral ligaments (HAGL), superior labral anteroposterior (SLAP) tears, capsular tears, and intra-articular incongruities [7]. However, MRI often underestimates the degree of glenoid-bone loss. Most traumatic glenohumeral instability is associated with soft tissue lesions, such as anteroinferior capsulolabral avulsion, and the typical finding is a Bankart lesion with or without capsular laxity [13, 14].

Tips and Tricks

- The West Point Axillary is the best plain radiograph for determining glenoid-bone loss, but it may be difficult to determine the exact amount without an advanced imaging study;
- a sagittal oblique MRI or MR arthrography (MRA) is helpful to assess glenoid-bone loss;
- a 3D CT scan sagittal oblique with the humeral head digitally subtracted is the gold standard for determining glenoid-bone loss.

6.5 Management and Surgical Decision Making

Nonsurgical management is indicated for patients with uncomplicated unidirectional traumatic instability [8]. Treatment consists of shoulder immobilization with a brace or harness to reduce capsular and labral lesions to their respective anatomic origins. A short period of immobilization is followed by range-of-motion exercise and physical therapy for rotator cuff and periscapular strengthening. Intensive physical therapy can be focused on scapular kinematics and proprioceptive training through biofeedback. Nonsurgical management may be preferred in elderly, debilitated patients with limited functional deficits and high potential surgical morbidity and mortality.

In general, surgical indications for open glenohumeral reconstruction are to restore the glenoid articular arc include failure of nonsurgical management, trauma, and recurrent episodes of glenohumeral instability evidenced by subluxation and dislocation; glenoid-bone loss >20%; a large (>30%) or engaging Hill-Sachs or Bankart lesion of the glenoid rim [4]; Instability Severity Index Score (ISIS) >6, and failed surgery for primary instability [8, 15]. The ISIS described by Balg and Boileau is based on a preoperative questionnaire, clinical exam, and review of X-rays [15]. Many decision algorithms for managing glenoid and humeral-head bone loss have been proposed, including one recently by Bollier and Arciero [16]. Young patients (<25 years) engaged in athletics or other high-demand activities may benefit from early surgical intervention, as may patients with significant bony injuries, rotator-cuff tears, or significant limitation in activities of daily living. Techniques for glenoid reconstruction include variations of the coracoid transfer [2, 3], iliac-crest autograft [4, 5], and distal tibia allograft, among others [6].

Although it is difficult to determine the exact level at which patients would benefit from an open glenoid-bone augmentation procedure, it has been suggested from both arthroscopic and open literature that glenoid defects >20–25% might be best suited for a primary open technique [17, 18]. A careful discussion with the patient is paramount to ascertain goals, desires, and return to sporting activity, as the open augmentation has been shown to have a lower rate of recurrent instability in certain high-level and functioning patient groups.

In this chapter, we outline the use of autologous intra-articular iliac-crest graft and distal tibia allograft for bony glenoid reconstruction for glenohumeral instability, indicating the key steps and pearls and pitfalls of each procedure.

6.6 Iliac-crest Graft Technique

Glenoid reconstruction using intra-articular bone graft with tricortical iliac-crest contoured to reestablish the concavity and width of the glenoid has been previously described [4, 5]. In this technique, the iliac crest graft is fixed with screws in combination with an anterior-inferior capsular repair to extend the anterior or posterior buttress of the glenoid to create a barrier for the humeral head. Iliac-crest graft reconstruction (particularly autograft) is a reliable method for grafting glenoid-bone defects and has shown good results in terms of functional scores, prevention of recurrent instability, excellent graft incorporation, and healing, with preservation of joint space [4, 5]. Auffarth et al. found no recurrences of instability and one traumatic graft failure using the iliac-crest bone-graft procedure in 47 patients with bony glenoid lesions [19]. Warner et al. demonstrated excellent outcomes in 11 patients with glenoid defects [5]. Iliac-crest autograft is a viable option given the nature of the autograft, ability to obtain large pieces of bone stock, and tricortical architecture of the graft.

6.6.1 Surgical Procedure

6.6.1.1 Patient Positioning

After induction of anesthesia using a regional block with or without general anesthesia, the patient is placed in the beach-chair position with the head of the bed elevated 40° and two small towels under the scapula (Fig. 6.1). Alternatively, the patient can be positioned supine with free arm movement or on a full-length beanbag with the head of the bed elevated to 30° and the ipsilateral iliac crest exposed. A beanbag is helpful to contour the patient to ensure that the shoulder is freely mobile and the iliac crest (contralateral iliac

Fig. 6.1. Patient in the beach-chair position with the head elevated 40°

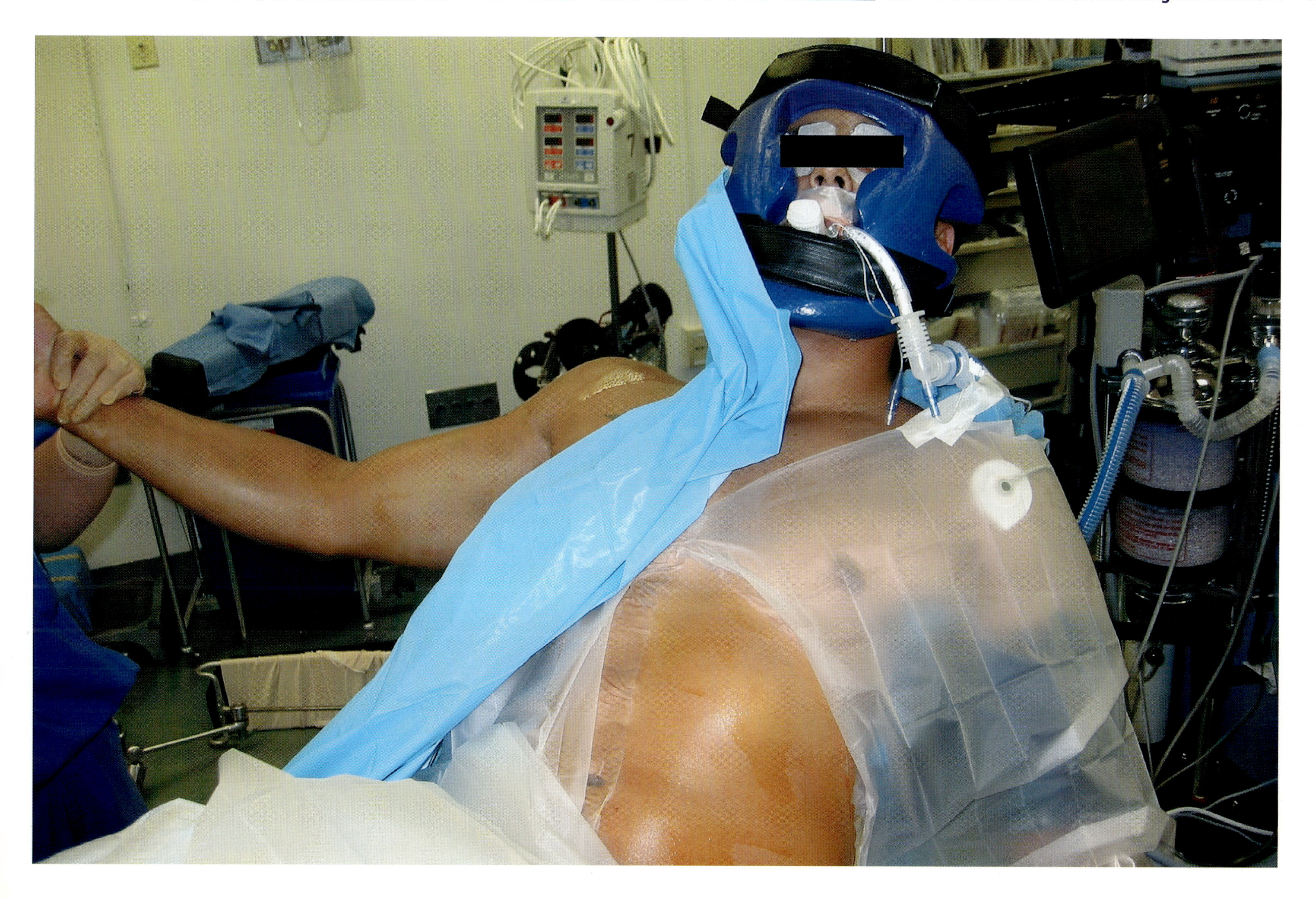

crest harvest is usually easiest) readily exposed. An examination under anesthesia is performed with the scapula stabilized to confirm the degree and direction of instability. The patient must be positioned in a manner that allows optimal visualization and screw trajectory. The surgical exposure uses the deltopectoral interval and extends from the coracoid to the axillary fold.

Tips and Tricks

- Place the patient in the beach-chair position and elevate the head of the bed to 30–40°;
- place two small towels under the medial border of the scapula to ensure the glenoid and scapula do not rotate anteriorly; this helps ensure that the drill for the glenoid screws is away from the patient's face;
- this positioning allows for optimal trajectory for working on the anterior aspect of the glenoid and easy screw-placement trajectory.

Complications

- Posterior rotation of the glenoid and difficulty with glenoid visualization;
- improper glenoid preparation and incorrect screw trajectory.

6.6.1.2 Incision and Approach

A standard anterior approach through the deltopectoral interval is performed. The incision extends from the coracoid to the superior tip of the axillary fold. The coracoid process and its muscle attachments, notably the short head of the biceps and coracobrachialis, are identified but not separated. Instead, they are gently retracted with a self-retaining retractor (Kolbel or equivalent) to protect the musculocutaneous nerve and obtain adequate exposure. The surgeon should ask the anesthesiologist for full muscle relaxation in instances where there is a difficult exposure or in particularly large patients, which will help make the procedure easier.

Tips and Tricks

- Take the cephalic vein laterally to avoid bleeding from the lateral branches;
- during the exposure, it is critical to palpate the axillary nerve;
- place a Kolbel retractor to retract the strap muscles;
- ask the anesthesiologist for full muscle relaxation.

Complications

- Injury to the axillary nerve due to stretching or laceration;
- injury to the musculocutaneous nerve located 5–8 cm distal to the coracoid insertion of the strap muscles.

6.6.1.3 Subscapularis Management

The subscapularis (SSc) tendon takedown is one of the most critical portions of this procedure. Inability to properly takedown and repair the SSc tendon can lead to atrophy of the SSc muscle and recurrent instability. The SSc tendon is identified and then can be handled in one of several ways: the upper two thirds may be taken down and the capsule identified medial to the SSc tendon insertion. Alternatively, the entire SSc tendon may be taken down, although many advocate maximal protection of the SSc tendon insertion on the humerus by performing an SSc tendon split in line with the fibers longitudinally. In this manner, the middle part of the tendon is sectioned longitudinally and the capsule identified medially. It should be noted that the nerve to the SSc muscle inserts anteriorly, about 1–2 cm medial to the coracoid, thus a medial longitudinal incision of the SSc tendon should not be taken medial to the coracoid.

Tips and Tricks

- The SSc tendon may either be split in line with the fibers or the top two thirds taken down. If possible, it is ideal to use a splitting approach to preserve the insertion on the humerus;
- when taking down the upper two thirds of the SSc tendon, the capsule can be delineated from the SSc tendon along its medial aspect (easier than laterally);
- use an elevator to tease the capsule from the SSc muscle, but only on the posterior aspect of the muscle to avoid the nerve, which penetrates anteriorly and 1 cm medial to the coracoid;
- elevate the capsule off the medial neck of the glenoid using a sharp elevator;
- elevate the capsule sharply off the glenoid neck; this is tagged and then repaired to the anterior aspect of the bone graft (usually with sutures placed under washers for the fixation screw);
- facilitate exposure with glenohumeral rotation and lateral traction.

Complications

- Iatrogenic injury to the nerve to the SSc muscle if capsule split made medial to the coracoid;
- inadequate glenoid visualization and thus improper graft placement;
- injury to the nerve to the SSc muscle, which penetrates the muscle anteriorly and 1 cm medial to the coracoid.

6.6.1.4 Glenoid Preparation

Once the SSc tendon is either longitudinally split or taken down (partial or full), the capsule is identified. The capsule is easiest to identify medial to the insertion, where it is less adherent to the tendon. The capsule is then released from the humeral neck and split down to the glenoid through the rotator interval region to create a capsulotomy at a 90° angle. This approach allows for more extensive visualization of the glenoid and increased mobilization of the capsule-periosteal sleeve from the anterior scapular neck. A periosteal elevator is used to elevate the capsule off the anterior glenoid neck to preserve as much capsular length as possible. Care is taken to avoid the axillary nerve with gentle digital protection. A blunt, curved retractor is then used to retract the soft tissues medially while a humeral-head retractor exposes the glenoid. It is critical to properly prepare the glenoid and achieve maximum exposure to determine the actual amount of missing glenoid. The length of the defect can be confirmed intraoperatively and compared with the preoperative measurement of glenoid-bone loss (Fig. 6.2). This measurement forms the basis for determining the size of the iliac-crest bone graft required for optimal reconstitution of the glenoid arc. A burr can be used to smooth the anterior glenoid, and an anterior glenoid retractor can be used to help attain adequate visualization. Generally, it is recommended not to overstuff the joint with bone but to reconstruct the anatomic glenoid size, adding in a few millimeters to ensure that there is adequate bone. At this point, the anterior portion of the native glenoid is prepared using a high-speed burr, rasp, and rongeur. Care is taken to preserve as much native glenoid bone as possible and to obtain a 90° angle to the face of the glenoid to accommodate the graft. In addition, the superior portion needs to be prepared in order to fit the graft without stepoff, and the overall glenoid-bone-loss interface is in line with the long axis of the glenoid. Final measurements after preparation confirm the size of iliac-crest harvest.

Tips and Tricks

- Use a small burr to create an even bleeding surface on the anterior glenoid; a long-barrel type burr is best to provide a flat and congruous surface;
- the amount of bone should be templated preoperatively; alternatively, take measurements using the bare spot as a marker to determine the amount of glenoid-bone loss.

Complications

- Improper glenoid preparation can lead to an uneven surface and potentially inadequate graft incorporation;
- soft tissue or axillary nerve can be wrapped up with the high-speed burr, so it is important to take care and use a retractor medial to the glenoid to decrease this risk;
- improper glenoid-bone-loss measurement can lead to inadequate graft placement.

Fig. 6.2. Preoperative computed tomography scan of the glenoid with 3D and digital subtraction of the humeral head prior to iliac-crest graft procedure

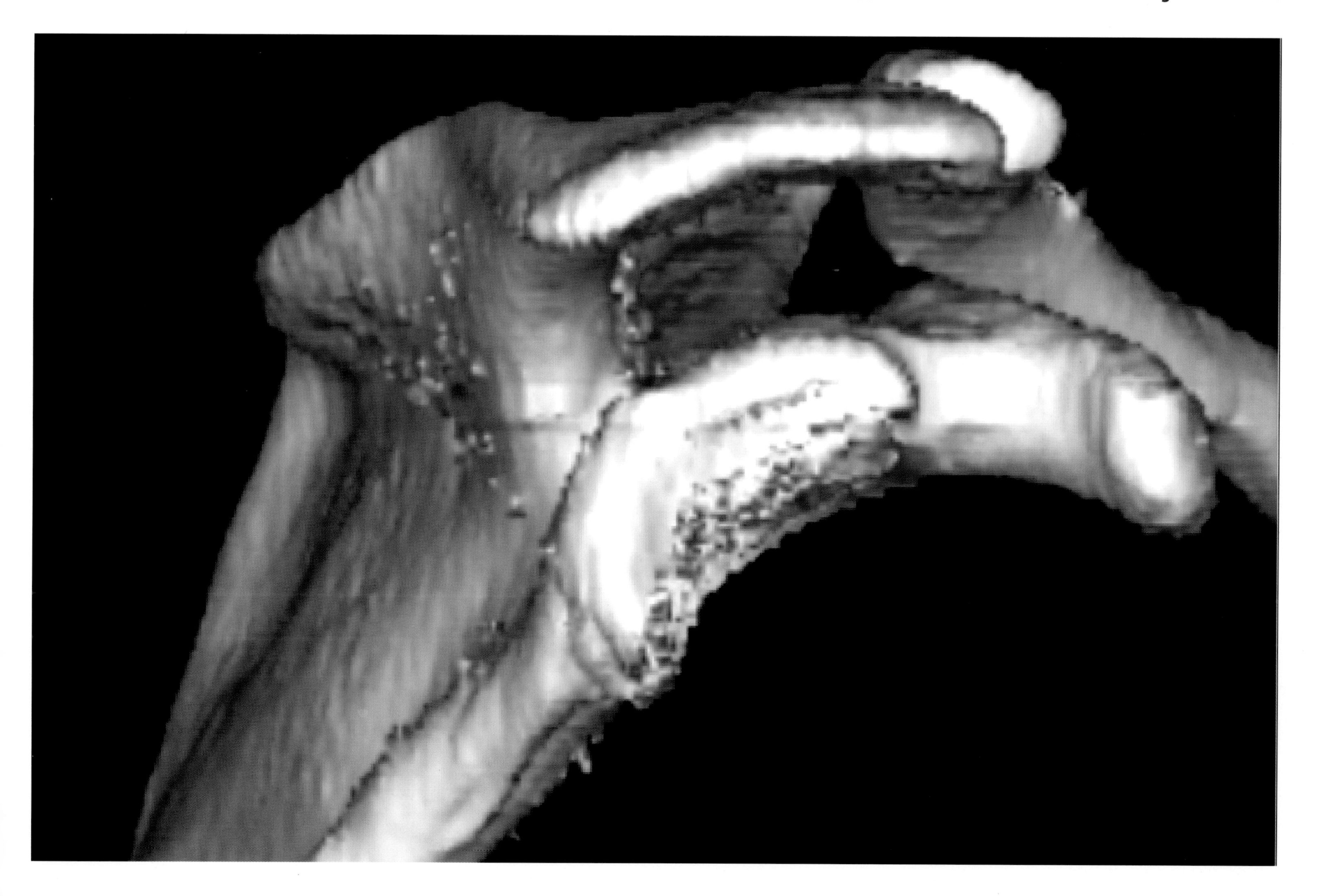

6.6.1.5 Iliac-crest Graft

The iliac crest is exposed with an incision posterior to the antero-superior iliac spine. The superior iliac crest is exposed with the inner and outer tables visualized, and blunt retractors are used to maintain exposure. Care is taken to ensure that the dissection is posterior to the anterior superior iliac spine (ASIS) to avoid the lateral femoral cutaneous nerve. An oscillating saw and osteotomes are used to remove a tricortical wedge-shaped graft that is generally 25- to 30-mm long by about 15-mm deep depending on the size of the glenoid defect. The periosteum over the defect is carefully closed in a watertight fashion, and skin is closed in layers. The inner table of the iliac crest is naturally concave and fits well on the glenoid to reconstitute the glenoid arc [20]. The iliac crest graft is contoured using a small saw and burr, and two holes are drilled in the graft for screw fixation so that it securely fits into the anterior glenoid. As the glenoid is prepared for the graft at a 90° angle to the glenoid surface, the deepest portion of the iliac crest is generally the face which comes in contact with the native glenoid, although other orientations of the graft have been described [5]. Regardless, the inner table of the iliac crest is best suited to become the glenoid face, as it has been shown that the inner surface most closely matches the contour of the native glenoid (Fig. 6.3) [20].

Tips and Tricks

- Use the periosteum that was dissected sharply off the iliac crest to close over the harvest site to decrease risk of hematoma and decrease postoperative pain;
- make the approach to the iliac crest from posterior to anterior to avoid injury to the lateral femoral cutaneous nerve across the ASIS;
- use either a small sagittal saw or osteotomes to make cuts in the inner and outer table.

Complications

- Lateral femoral cutaneous nerve injury when dissecting across the anterior superior iliac spine.
- fracture to the iliac crest with improper cuts and depth of cut.

Fig. 6.3. Iliac-crest graft placement to the anterior glenoid

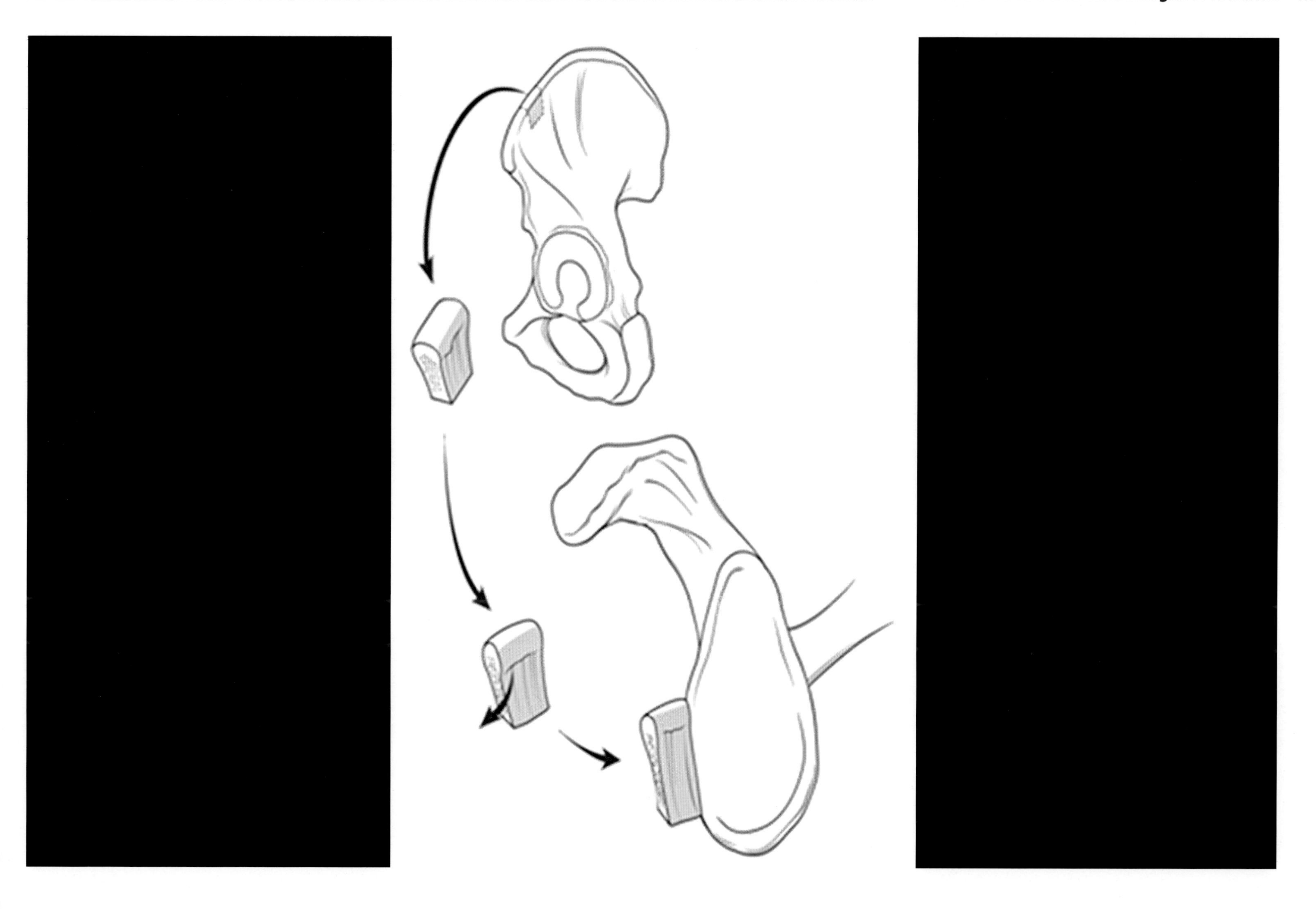

6.6.1.6 Iliac-crest Graft Placement and Closure

Once the graft is appropriately contoured to match the desired dimensions and fit, it is temporarily fixed in place using two to three small 1.5-mm Kirschner (K) wires and 3.5-mm noncannulated or 4.0-mm cannulated screws with washers. Typically, the K wires are placed and oriented medially and parallel to the joint surface so that the screw heads sit medially and away from the humeral articular surface. A no. 2 nonabsorbable suture is placed underneath the washer before complete seating so that the suture remains well attached after fixation (Fig. 6.4). This suture becomes an anchor that is used to repair the labrum and capsule-periosteal sleeve to the edge of the iliac-crest graft. The capsule-periosteal sleeve is then repaired to the anterior edge of the graft using horizontal mattress sutures with no. 2 braided suture fixed underneath each screw washer. If the capsule cannot be reattached to the neck of the humerus with the arm in at least 30° of external rotation, the lateral portion of the SSc tendon can be used as an extension of the capsule so that the capsule is tensioned in external rotation. Thus, the iliac-crest bone graft becomes an intra-articular graft with the capsular complex affixed to the anterior aspect of the graft. A drain may be placed under the deltoid prior to closure. The incision is closed in layers with a 1-0 Vicryl suture to reapproximate the deltopectoral interval, subcutaneous resorbable 2-0 monofilament, and subcuticular 3-0 running monofilament suture with Steristrips. The incision is then dressed with sterile bandages and the shoulder placed into a shoulder immobilizer with an abduction wedge. The shoulder immobilizer should be kept on for 4 weeks, with pendulum exercises and passive forward flexion and external rotation range of motion initiated after the first week. After 4 weeks, the patients may begin supervised physical therapy to regain motion and may return to activities of daily living. Strengthening and conditioning exercise are allowed after 3 months, and overhead activities and noncontact recreational sports are allowed after 4 months. A postoperative CT scan to visualize proper alignment and incorporation of the

Fig. 6.4. Iliac-crest graft fixation with 3.5-mm noncannulated screws with washers. A no. 2 nonabsorbable suture is placed under the washers to function as suture anchors to repair the labrum and capsule-periosteal sleeve to the edge of the graft

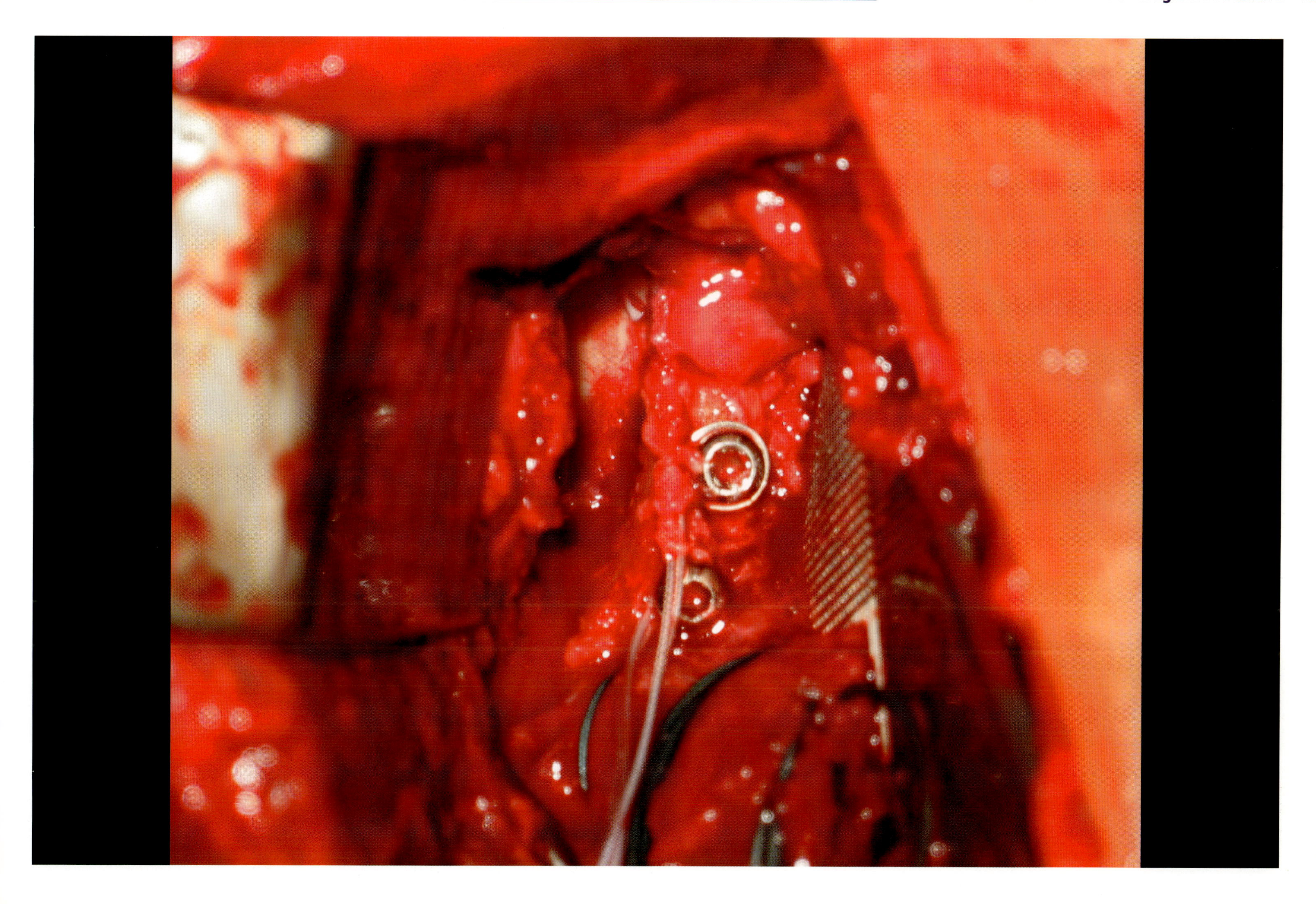

iliac-crest graft may be obtained several months after surgery during routine follow-up (Fig. 6.5).

Tips and Tricks

- Use the inner table of the iliac-crest graft to match the glenoid face; this is concave and fits the glenoid well [20]
- either predrilled two holes spaced approximately 5- to 7-mm apart into the graft for screw fixation or place K wires and affix temporarily wires and then drill with a long 2.5-mm bit with a drill guide in place;
- use two 3.5-mm, noncannulated, fully threaded cortical screws to affix graft with small washers;
- place a no. 2 nonabsorbable suture underneath the washer to function as a suture anchor for labral and capsular fixation;
- repair capsule to the anterior edge of the graft, with the sutures underneath the washers;
- a suture anchor can be placed at the 6-o'clock position of the glenoid and used to help achieve capsular closure;
- repair the capsule with the arm in at least 30° of external rotation to avoid external rotation loss.

Complications

- Pre-drilling of the two screw holes at an improper angle can lead to improper screw tract into the glenoid;
- holes must not be drilled too close to each other, as this can lead to the inability to place two screws into the graft;
- keep screws deep to the glenoid surface so the washers do not articulate on the humeral head.

Fig. 6.5. Postoperative 3D reconstruction computed tomography scan showing proper alignment and incorporation of the iliac-crest graft into the glenoid

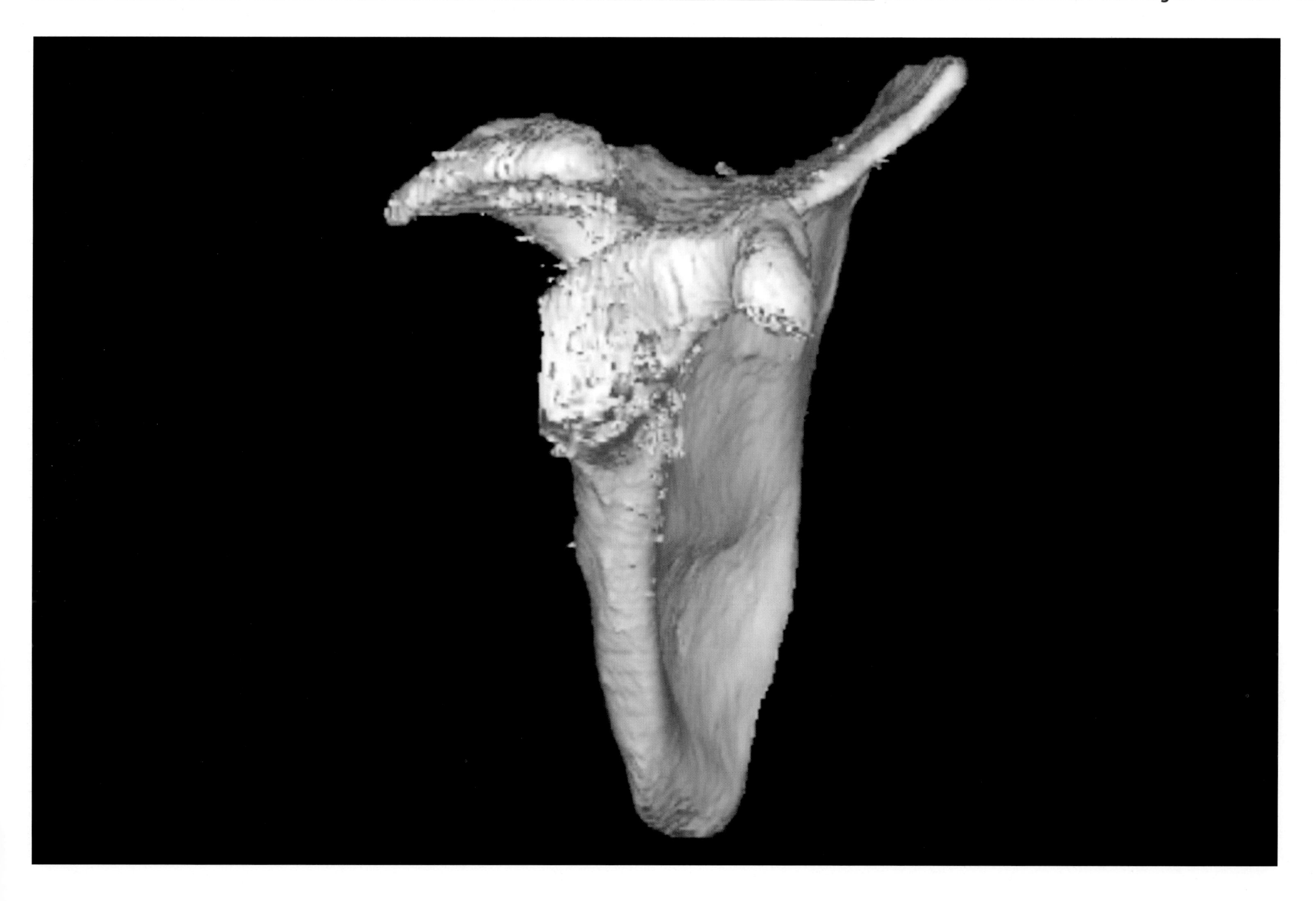

6.7 Distal Tibia Allograft Technique

The vast majority of bone grafting techniques for glenoid-bone loss are bony solutions without cartilage reconstitution. Although fresh glenoid allograft has been described, it is difficult to obtain due to infection concerns, harvesting techniques, and donor factors. To identify alternate sources of osteochondral grafting options for the glenoid, we found the distal lateral aspect of the tibia nearly matches the curvature and concavity of the native glenoid [6]. Fresh distal tibia allografts are more readily available than fresh glenoid allografts secondary to decreased risk of contamination (the glenoid is closer to the core of the body during harvest and has a higher chance of contamination), as well as better availability from donor companies due to graft-harvest techniques and preservation of the donated cadaver.

One of the main advantages of the distal tibia is that it contains dense weight-bearing corticocancellous bone with a cartilaginous surface that nearly matches the native curvature of the glenoid [6], allowing excellent screw fixation and host-graft incorporation. Distal tibia allograft avoids the potential donor-site morbidity associated with coracoid transfer and nonanatomic placement of the conjoined tendon [21–23]. It also permits restoration of the articular surface of the glenoid with robust weight-bearing cartilage and the ability to provide an anatomic fit by customizing the graft size for the individual defect. However, there are the potential concerns of fresh allograft incorporation, possible mismatch, and bony resorption. To date, the first author has performed 14 such allografts: 13 patients went back to full duty, and all 14 patients presented proper incorporation of the fresh allograft bone at 2 years of follow-up. Another benefit of the technique is that the distal tibia graft curvature radius is nearly identical to that of the glenoid, with a well-matched cartilage thickness.

6.7.1 Surgical Procedure

6.7.1.1 Patient Positioning

After induction of anesthesia using a regional block with or without general anesthesia, the patient is placed in the beach-chair position with the head elevated 40°. Two sterile towels are placed behind the medial border of the scapula on the operative shoulder between the patient and the bed to ensure that the glenoid and scapula do not rotate anteriorly. This positioning ensures optimal trajectory for working on the anterior aspect of the glenoid and allows easy trajectory of screw fixation for the fresh distal tibia allograft later in the procedure.

6.7.1.2 Incision and Approach

Overall glenoid exposure and preparation are similar to those for the iliac-crest technique. Once the anterior glenoid is identified, the amount of glenoid-bone loss can be confirmed against preoperative imaging (Fig. 6.6). If there is 25–30% of glenoid-bone loss, this indicates that ~8 to 9 mm of anterior glenoid bone will be needed for allograft augmentation; however, it is acceptable to use more bone than is required to reconstitute the loss.

Fig. 6.6. Preoperative computed tomography scan of the glenoid with 3D and digital subtraction of the humeral head prior to distal tibia allograft procedure showing ~35% anterior glenoid-bone loss

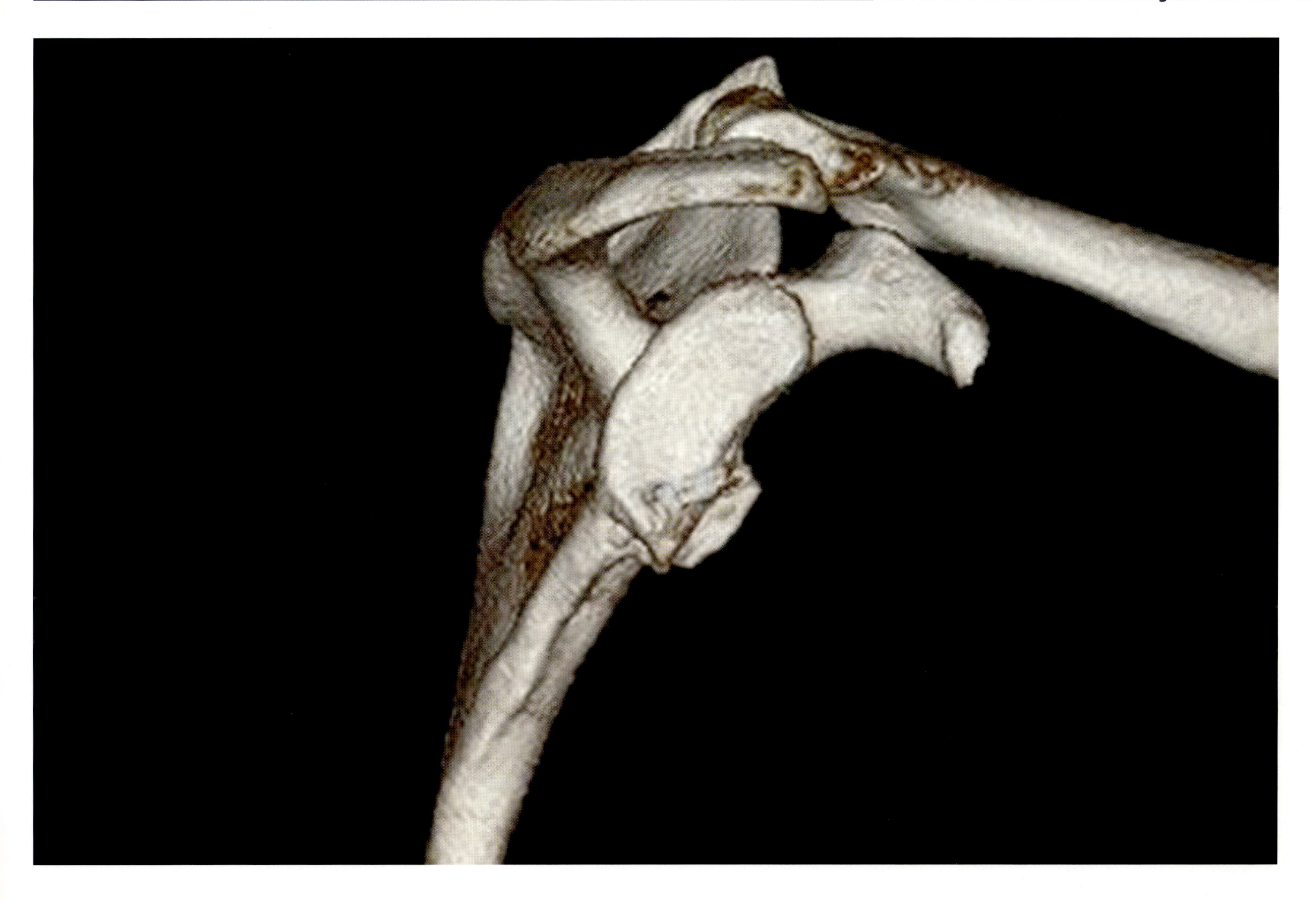

6.7.1.3 Anterior Glenoid Preparation

The anterior glenoid is then prepared. Any remaining labral tissue is elevated and dissected medially, with care taken to protect the axillary nerve located directly inferiorly. The labrum may be preserved and eventually repaired to the anterior aspect of the allograft, with sutures affixed to the screws. Occasionally, the anterior labrum is deficient, especially in revision surgery, and not amenable to repair. A combination of a high-speed burr, rasp, and curette is used to create a surface perpendicular to the glenoid cartilage face in order to accommodate the fresh distal tibia bone graft. A high-speed bur is used on the anterior aspect of the glenoid in the area of the defect to refine a uniform surface perpendicular to the glenoid articular surface to accommodate the distal tibia allograft. Measurements of the amount of bone loss based on the bare spot are confirmed prior to allograft preparation (Fig. 6.7) [24].

Fig. 6.7. Intraoperative measurement of glenoid-bone loss to determine amount of distal tibia allograft required for augmentation

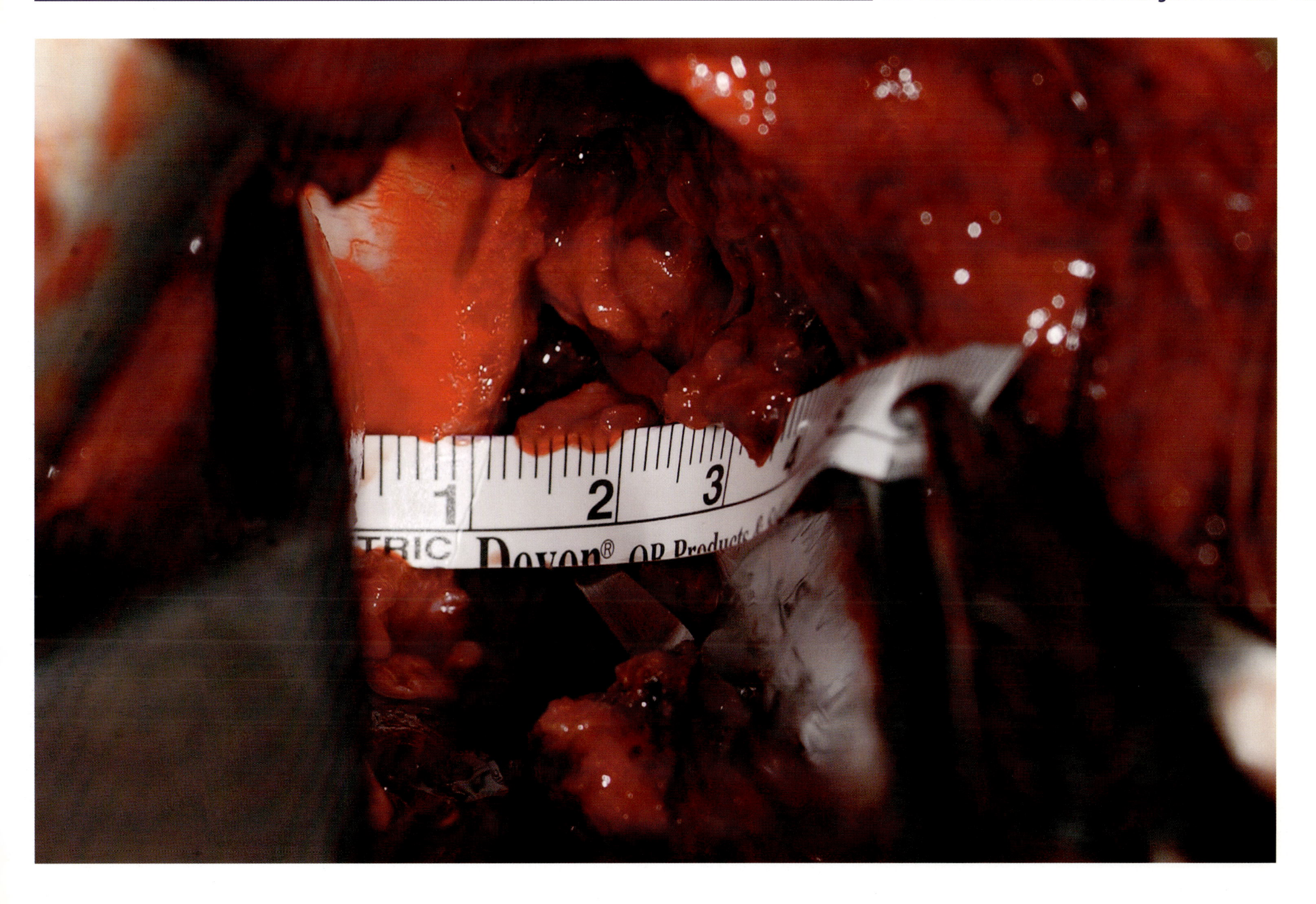
1
2
3
Devon®

6.7.1.4 *Distal Tibia Allograft Preparation*

Fresh distal tibia allograft is obtained from a cadaveric donor source using good-practice harvesting techniques. The distal tibia is stored in sterile medium and transported to the operating room without freezing. The lateral one third of the distal tibia is used for the graft and measurements are confirmed from preoperative CT scan and intraoperative measurements. The distal tibia is marked, and cuts are made with a thin 0.5-in. sagittal saw while an assistant holds the graft in place with two towel clamps to reduce movement (Fig. 6.8a-c). Irrigation is used to keep the allograft cool and avoid thermal injury while making the cuts. To accommodate any slope changes of the glenoid, the allograft may be cut at various angles. Typically, between 8 and 11 mm of tibia bone measured on the articular surface is used, depending on the glenoid defect size and severity. The graft is then cut to fit a superior-to-inferior size of approximately

Fig. 6.8a-c. **a** Lateral aspect of the distal tibia is used as the graft source. Preparation of the distal tibia allograft with marks and cuts for 8-mm deficiency as seen from the bottom; **b** front of the graft; **c** the graft is cut to accommodate the perpendicular cut to the glenoid surface

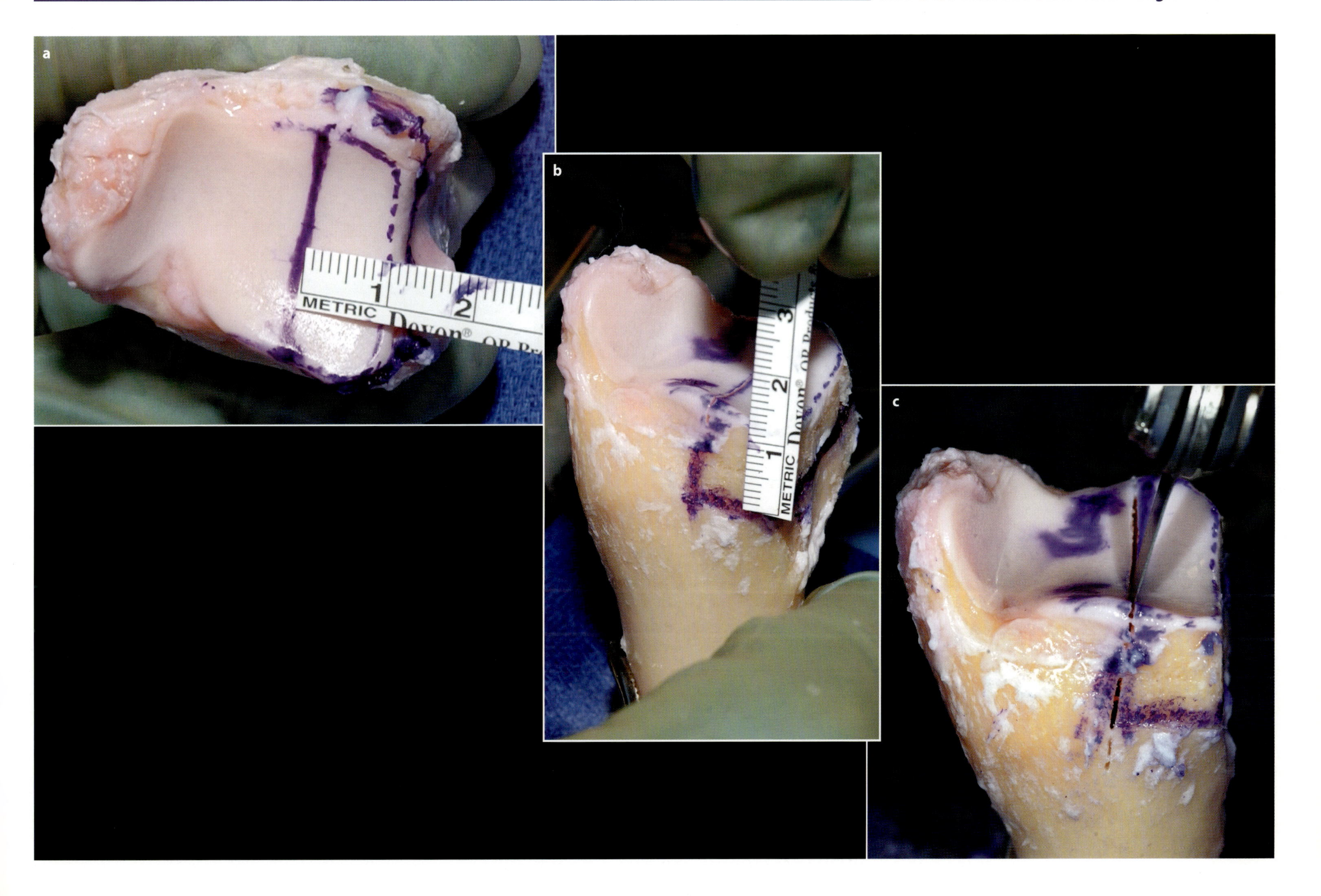
a
METRIC
b
METRIC
Devon®
c

25–28 mm and approximately 10–15 mm deep (medially on the glenoid) (Fig. 6.9a, b).

Tips and Tricks

- Towel clamps or a graft holder is used to stabilize the graft;
- a 0.5-mm ×10-mm-wide sagittal saw is best to make fine cuts;
- irrigation is used to keep graft cool while cutting;
- glenoid interface cut angle (the one most medial on the tibia) is about 10–15° to accommodate the natural curvature on the glenoid (slightly up anteriorly);
- pulse lavage irrigation is performed after the graft is fashioned to wash away marrow elements;
- two 1.25-mm K wires are placed in at a slight angle to facilitate passage, placement, and temporary fixation;
- two 3.5-mm fully threaded cortical screws are used to fix the graft; "lag" technique may be used with slight over-drilling of the outer cortex with a 3.5-mm drill to allow for graft compression;
- washers are placed under the screws with no. 2 nonabsorbable suture to repair the medially elevated glenohumeral capsule.

Complications

- Improper graft cut can lead to difficulty with placement on the anterior glenoid surface;
- improper screw placement can lead to inability to place graft accurately along prepared glenoid surface;
- screw sizes >36–40 mm could potentially exit posterior to the glenoid and cause nerve damage.

Fig. 6.9a, b. **a** Final width; **b** length of the distal tibia allograft. The graft is cut to fit the superior-to-inferior size of the glenoid defect with a depth matching that of the medial glenoid

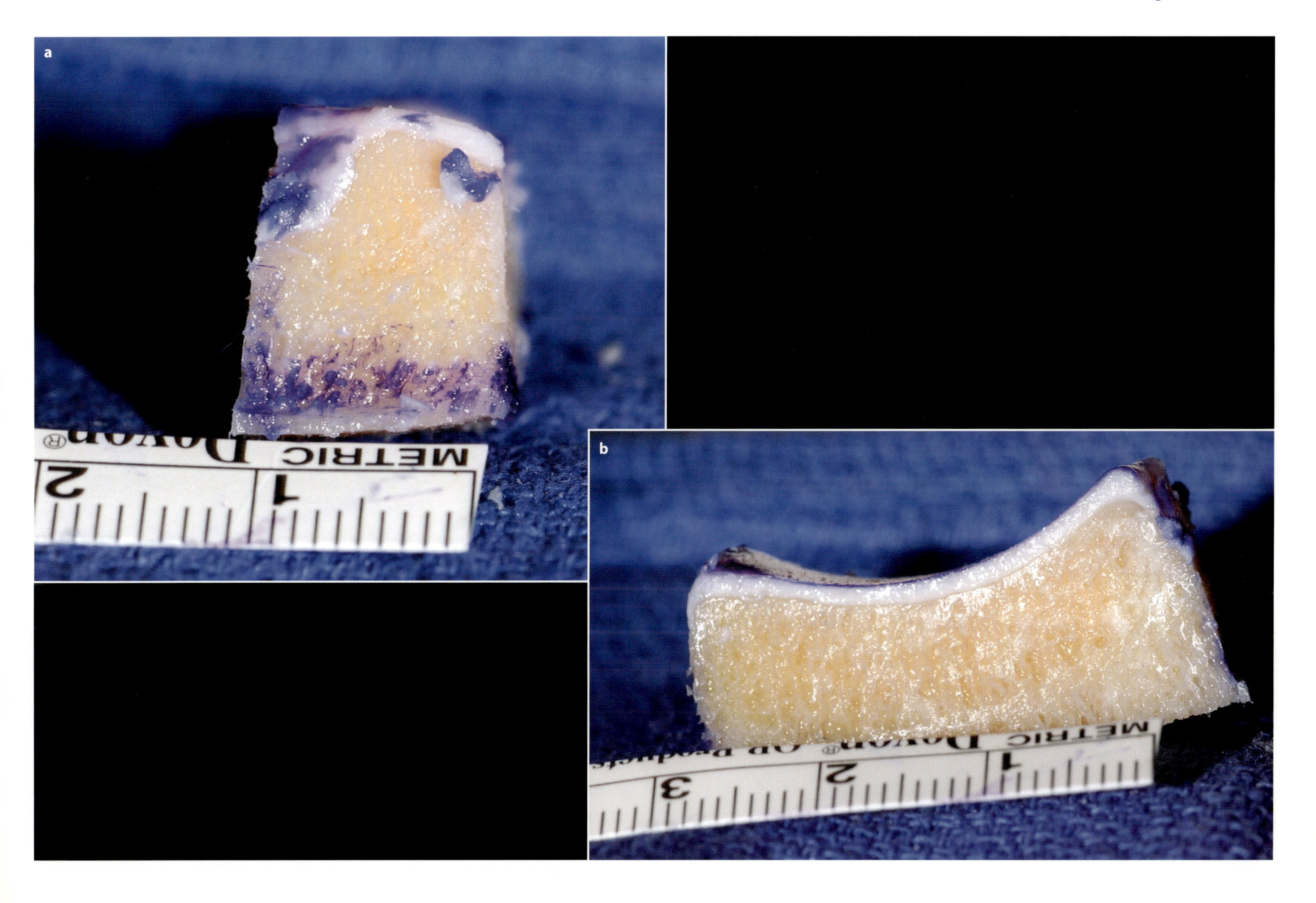
a
b

6.7.1.5 *Distal Tibia Allograft Placement and Closure*

The most superior and inferior aspects of the distal tibia allograft are rounded to a glenoid shape using a small sagittal saw; two 1.6-mm K wires are placed in the allograft bone at a 45° angle to the articular surface to facilitate placement and positioning within the joint (Fig. 6.10). The allograft is then transferred to the native glenoid to assess fit, conformity, and angle relative to the articular surface. Additional cuts can be made to improve graft conformity. Once graft-fit is confirmed, the two small 1.6-mm

Fig. 6.10. Two 1.6-mm Kirschner (K) wires are placed in the tibia allograft at a 45° angle to the glenoid surface to facilitate positioning in the glenoid

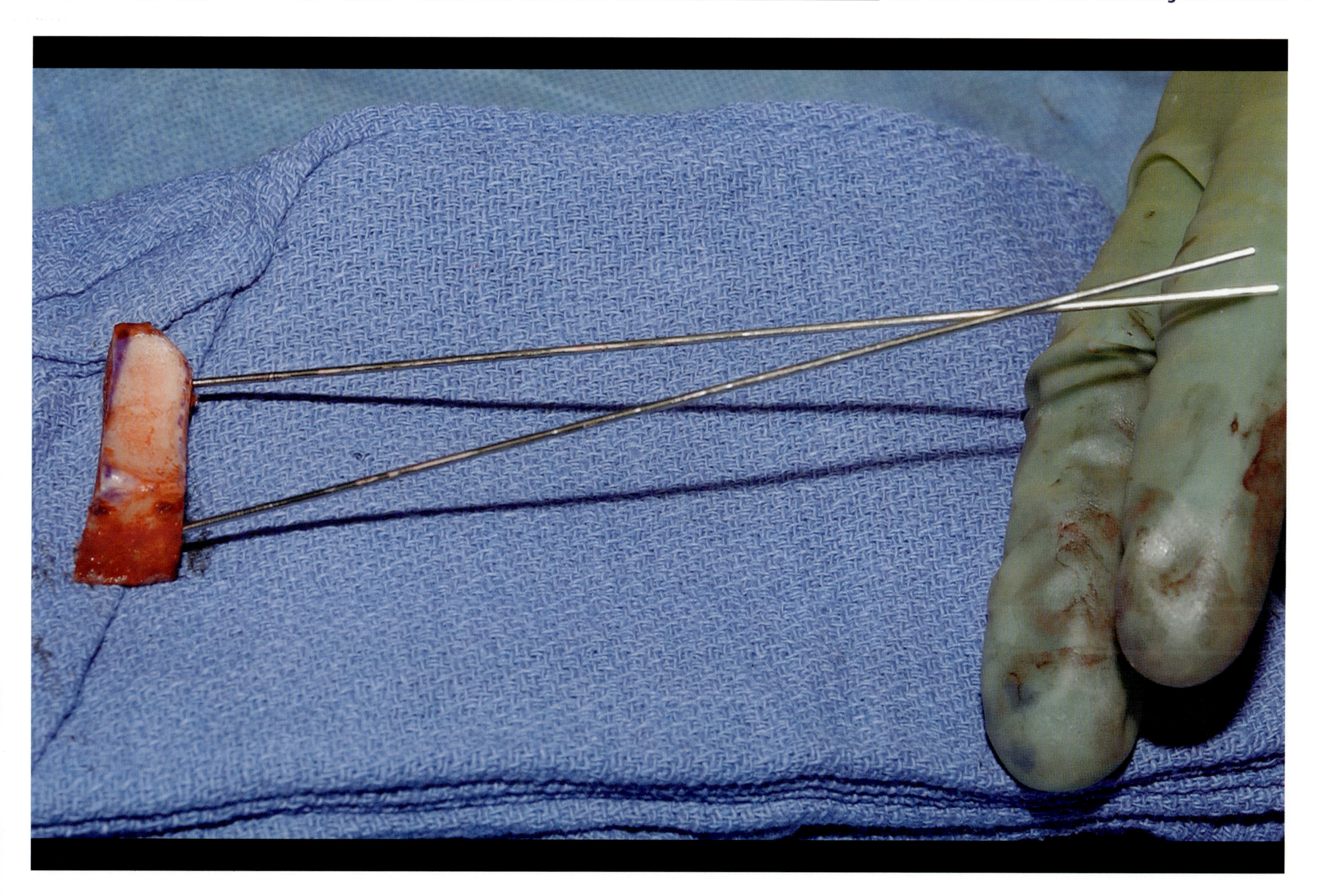

K wires previously placed are drilled into the native glenoid to temporarily affix the graft (Fig. 6.11). The graft may need to be slightly adjusted, but it is important to place the graft in the inferior two thirds of the glenoid, as this is where the humerus articulates, and it is the important position to prevent recurrent anterior instability. Depending on defect size, for a 20–30% glenoid-bone loss, the graft generally measures approximately 25–30 mm of bone from superior to inferior, 7–10 mm anterior to posterior, and about 10–12 mm lateral to medial (depth). The graft is then fixed with two 3.5-mm fully threaded cortical screws between 32 and 40 mm long using a lag technique for compression and a small washer (Fig. 6.12). If the capsule and labrum are available for repair, they are then stitched back down with suture that was placed underneath the washers before final tightening. The SSc tendon is then closed with standard techniques using tendon-bone fixation or side-to-side repair (for split SSc tendon approach) and approximation with no. 2 nonabsorbable suture, and the remaining closure is completed. A drain is then placed underneath the deltoid and tucked into the lateral recess. A drain may be omitted if the deep wound is dry.

Fig. 6.11. Once allograft positioning is confirmed in the glenoid, the two attached Kirschner (K) wires are drilled into the native glenoid for temporary fixation

Fig. 6.12. Once final positioning is confirmed, the graft is fixed with two 3.5-mm fully threaded cortical screws between 32- and 38-mm long with a small washer

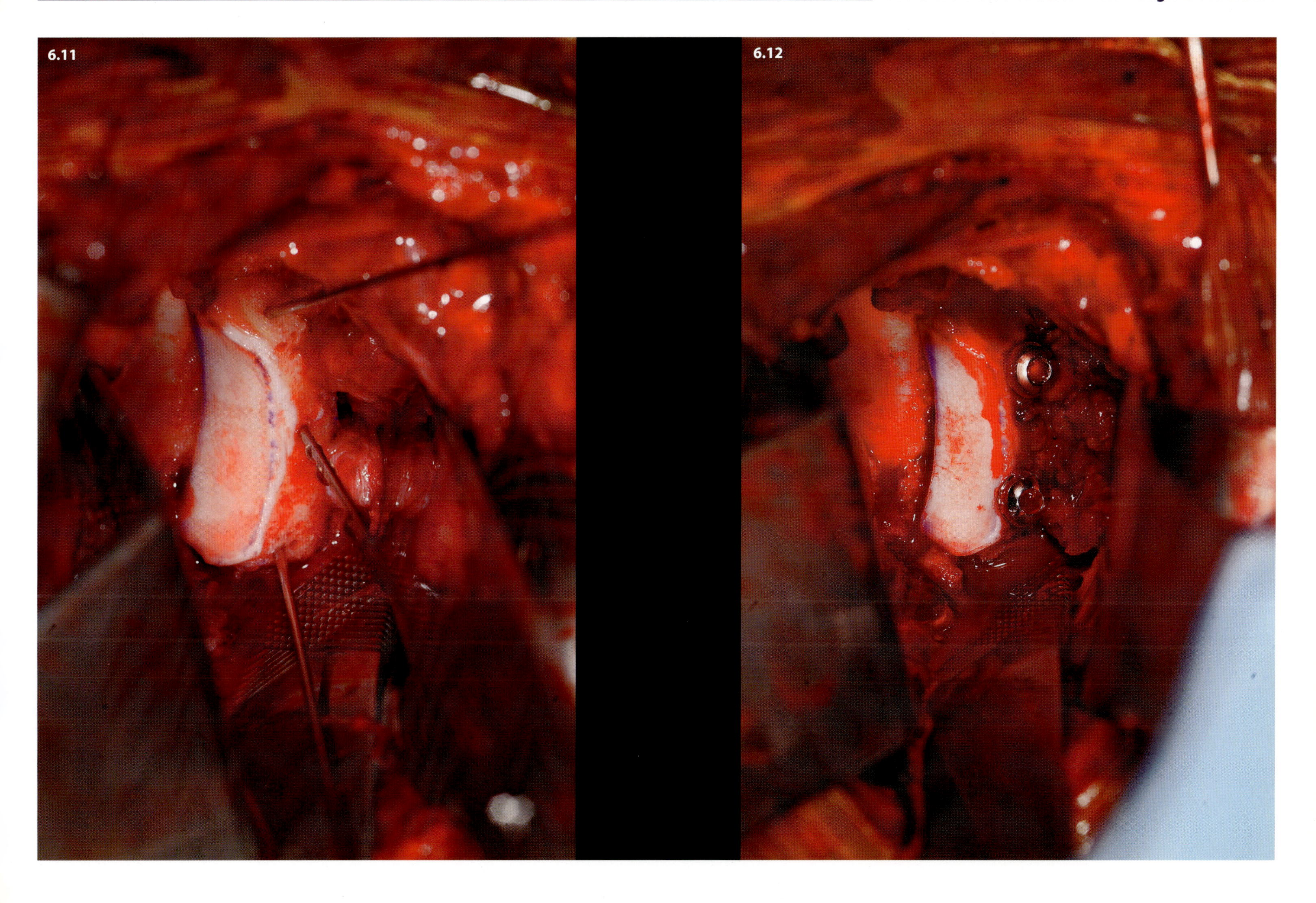
6.11
6.12

Postoperatively, the patient's extremity is placed in a shoulder immobilizer abduction sling. The patient undergoes pendulum exercises and passive range of motion in the scapular plane (90° forward flexion, 30° external rotation) with active range of motion of the elbow, wrist, and hand for the first 4 weeks. At 4 weeks, active assisted exercises are instituted, followed by more active range-of-motion exercises by 6–8 weeks. At 6 weeks, the sling is removed and additional stretching followed by a strengthening program is initiated, followed by return to full activity in 4–6 months, depending on successful graft incorporation, functional range of motion, and strength recovery. A postoperative CT scan may be obtained to view final distal tibia allograft orientation and incorporation into the glenoid (Fig. 6.13).

Fig. 6.13. Postoperative 3D reconstruction computed tomography scan showing orientation and incorporation of the distal tibia allograft into the glenoid with reconstitution of the glenoid articular arc

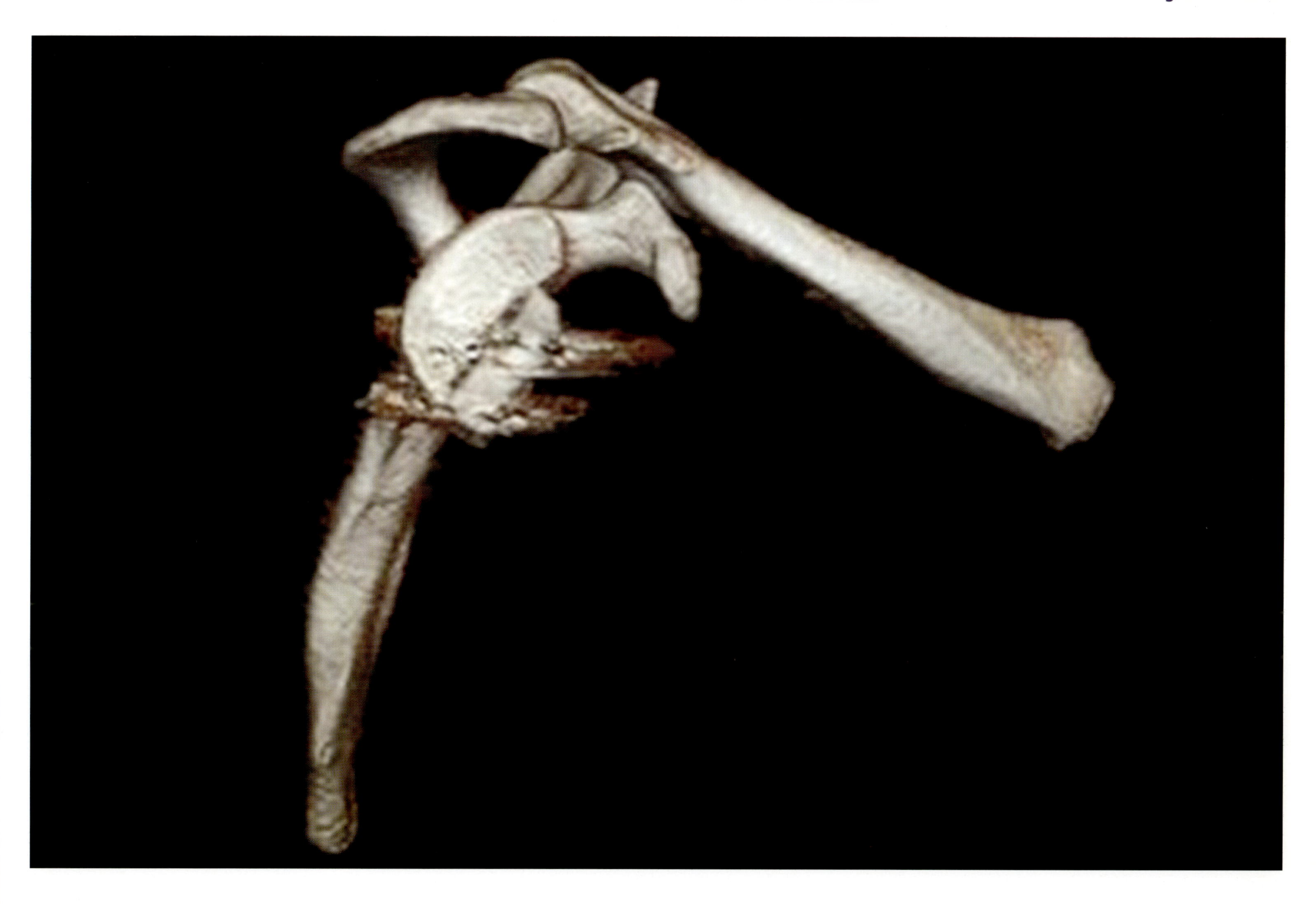

References

1. Canale SB, JH (2007) Campbell's Operative Orthopaedics, 11th edn. Mosby, St. Louis
2. Hovelius L, Sandstrom B, Sundgren K et al (2004) One hundred eighteen Bristow-Latarjet repairs for recurrent anterior dislocation of the shoulder prospectively followed for fifteen years: study I-clinical results. J Shoulder Elbow Surg 13:509-516
3. Schroder DT, Provencher MT, Mologne TS et al (2006) The modified Bristow procedure for anterior shoulder instability: 26-year outcomes in Naval Academy midshipmen. Am J Sports Med 34:778-786
4. Haaker RG, Eickhoff U, and Klammer HL (1993) Intraarticular autogenous bone grafting in recurrent shoulder dislocations. Mil Med 158:164-169
5. Warner JJ, Gill TJ, O'Hollerhan J D et al (2006) Anatomical glenoid reconstruction for recurrent anterior glenohumeral instability with glenoid deficiency using an autogenous tricortical iliac crest bone graft. Am J Sports Med 34:205-212
6. Provencher MT, Ghodadra N, LeClere L et al (2009) Anatomic osteochondral glenoid reconstruction for recurrent glenohumeral instability with glenoid deficiency using a distal tibia allograft. Arthroscopy 25:446-452
7. Arciero RA, Spang JT (2008) Complications in arthroscopic anterior shoulder stabilization: pearls and pitfalls. Instr Course Lect 57:113-124
8. Schepsis A, Busconi B eds (2006) Orthopaedic surgery essentials, Lippincott Williams & Wilkins, Philadelphia
9. Schenk TJ, Brems JJ (1998) Multidirectional instability of the shoulder: pathophysiology, diagnosis, and management. J Am Acad Orthop Surg 6:65-72
10. Itoi E, Lee SB, Amrami KK et al (2003) Quantitative assessment of classic anteroinferior bony Bankart lesions by radiography and computed tomography. Am J Sports Med 31:112-118
11. Griffith JF, Antonio GE, Tong CW et al (2003) Anterior shoulder dislocation: quantification of glenoid bone loss with CT. AJR Am J Roentgenol 180:1423-1430
12. Sugaya H, Moriishi J, Dohi M et al (2003) Glenoid rim morphology in recurrent anterior glenohumeral instability. J Bone Joint Surg Am 85:878-884
13. Apreleva M, Hasselman CT, Debski RE et al (1998) A dynamic analysis of glenohumeral motion after simulated capsulolabral injury. A cadaver model. J Bone Joint Surg Am 80:474-480
14. Bigliani LU, Pollock RG, Soslowsky LJ et al (1992) Tensile properties of the inferior glenohumeral ligament. J Orthop Res 10:187-197
15. Balg F, Boileau P (2007) The instability severity index score. A simple pre-operative score to select patients for arthroscopic or open shoulder stabilisation. J Bone Joint Surg Br 89:1470-1477
16. Bollier MJ, Arciero R (2010) Management of glenoid and humeral bone loss. Sports Med Arthrosc 18:140-148
17. Boileau P, Villalba M, Hery JY et al (2006) Risk factors for recurrence of shoulder instability after arthroscopic Bankart repair. J Bone Joint Surg Am 88:1755-1763
18. Mologne TS, Provencher MT, Menzel KA et al (2007) Arthroscopic stabilization in patients with an inverted pear glenoid: results in patients with bone loss of the anterior glenoid. Am J Sports Med 35:1276-1283
19. Auffarth A, Schauer J, Matis N et al (2008) The J-bone graft for anatomical glenoid reconstruction in recurrent posttraumatic anterior shoulder dislocation. Am J Sports Med 36:638-647
20. Ghodadra N, Gupta A, Romeo AA et al (2010) Normalization of glenohumeral articular contact pressures after Latarjet or iliac crest bone-grafting. J Bone Joint Surg Am 92:1478-1489
21. Burkhart SS, De Beer JF (2000) Traumatic glenohumeral bone defects and their relationship to failure of arthroscopic Bankart repairs: significance of the inverted-pear glenoid and the humeral engaging Hill-Sachs lesion. Arthroscopy 16:677-694
22. Hovelius LK, Sandstrom BC, Rosmark DL et al (2001) Long-term results with the Bankart and Bristow-Latarjet procedures: recurrent shoulder instability and arthropathy. J Shoulder Elbow Surg 10:445-452
23. Pagnani MJ (2008) Open capsular repair without bone block for recurrent anterior shoulder instability in patients with and without bony defects of the glenoid and/or humeral head. Am J Sports Med 36:1805-1812
24. Lo IK, Parten PM, and Burkhart SS (2004) The inverted pear glenoid: an indicator of significant glenoid bone loss. Arthroscopy 20:169-174

Chapter 7 – Treating Recurrent Anterior Glenohumeral Instability Using an Autogenous Tricortical Iliac-crest Bone Graft: Eden-hybbinette Procedure

Dario Petriccioli, Celeste Bertone and Giacomo Marchi

7.1 Introduction

Traumatic anterior instability is one of the most commonly diagnosed and treated conditions of the shoulder and is often associated with bone loss from the glenoid, the humerus, or both. It is recognized that bony defects of the anterior glenoid are common among shoulders with recurrent instability [1, 2]. A significant glenoid bone defect limits the effectiveness of arthroscopic repair of anteroinferior shoulder instability [3]. The critical size of the defect above which an arthroscopic Bankart repair becomes ineffective has been estimated by Itoi et al. [4] to be an average width of 6.8 mm, or 21% of the glenoid length. In defects of this size, the translational force required to subluxate the humeral head in abduction and external rotation is significantly decreased. If a critical bony glenoid defect is not addressed along with arthroscopic capsulolabral refixation, the risk of redislocation is increased, resulting in recurrence rates reported to range from 56% to 67% [4]. Yamamoto et al. confirmed that an osseous defect width 19% of the glenoid length remains unstable even after Bankart-lesion repair [5].

We use 3D reconstructed computed tomography (CT) scans with humeral-head subtraction using the Proven Excellence Biograph Duo LSO (Pico) system to compare with the contralateral healthy side to more accurately quantify glenoid-defect size to define surgical planning [6]. Lesions are classified as small (<5%), medium (5–20%), large (>20%), and massive (>30%). When surgery is considered for recurrent anterior glenohumeral instability, we not only identify the mechanical problem of instability but also perform a careful assessment of the patient and any comorbid conditions, such as epilepsy, rotator-cuff deficiency, and multidirectional instability associated with generalized ligament laxity.

In our practice, arthroscopic Bankart repair is the primary treatment for refractory anterior instability with small glenoid-bone defect or one of medium size in elderly, low-activity-demand patients. We use an open technique (Latarjet procedure) when the bone loss appears to have approached 20–25% (large defect) of the surface area of the native glenoid or when the impression injury to the humeral head appears to engage the anterior glenoid rim within a functional arc of motion. Generally, defects involving approximately 30% or more of the glenoid articular surface are treated with open bone grafting (autograft or allograft) [7–11]. The use of structural bone grafting to reconstruct the anterior-inferior glenoid is referred to as the Eden-Hybbinette procedure, as anterior glenoid grafting was first described in 1918 by Eden [12] and in 1932 by Hybbinette [13]. The procedure was first performed using tibial autograft. In our practice, the procedure consists of a tricortical iliac-crest bone graft fixed to the anterior glenoid neck using 4.5-mm screws [14–17].

7.2 Surgical Technique

7.2.1 Patient Positioning

As shown in Fig. 7.1, the procedure is performed with the patient under general endotracheal anesthesia combined with an anterior

Fig. 7.1. Patient positioning: modified beach-chair position

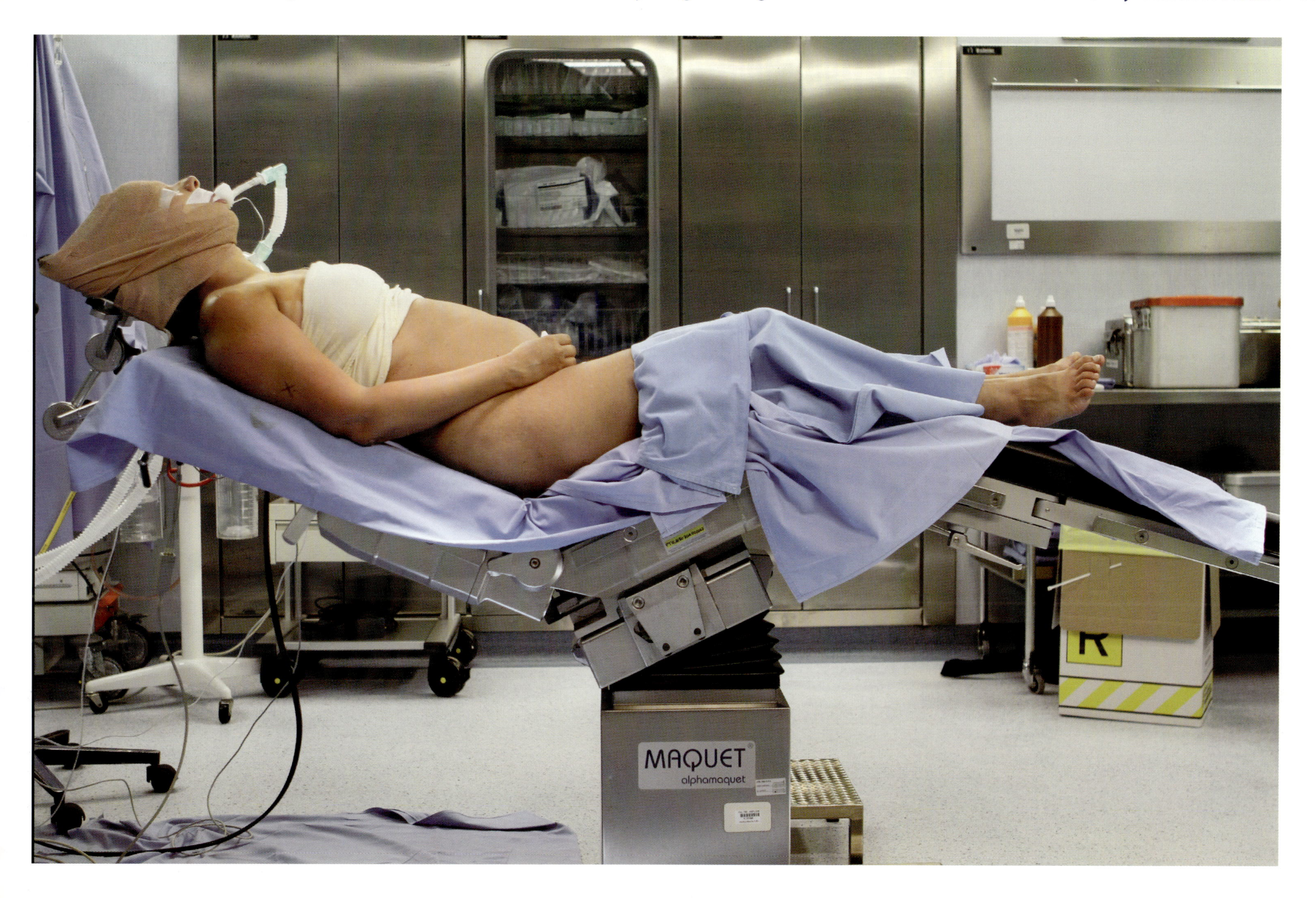
MAQUET
alphamaquet

interscalene cervical plexus block. The patient is placed in a modified beach-chair position on the edge of a standard operating table that allows for flexion of approximately 45° at the waist and 30° of flexion at the knees to prevent the patient from sliding distally. The entire arm should be draped and freely movable. For this reason, it is helpful to use an operating table specifically designed for shoulder surgery that includes a removable lateral portion expose the shoulder girdle for the requisite intraoperative shoulder positioning. The ipsilateral anterior iliac crest is also prepared and draped for the bone-graft harvest.

Tips and Tricks

Placing a pillow under the patient's knees helps maintain the flexed position and avoids pressure on nerves.

Complications

Malpositioning can lead to significant upper- and lower-extremity neurapraxias as well as soft-tissue injury away from the surgical site.

7.2.2 Deltopectoral Approach: Incision

We consider the deltopectoral approach as the standard approach for anterior shoulder stabilization. With the arm abducted (Fig. 7.2), the skin incision is marked off with an indelible pencil starting slightly medial to the coracoid and extending 5 cm distally parallel to the anterior margin of the deltoid muscle. Sharp dissection through the subcutaneous tissues extends to the deltoid fascia.

Tips and Tricks

The subcutis must be undermined extensively, particularly laterally and cranially, as far as the tip of the coracoid process, thus allowing the surgical field to be displaced upward by several centimeters with a Hohmann retractor over the coracoid process.

Complications

The subsequent scar can be a cosmetic concern for many patients. Placing the incision more lateral to the anterior axillary fold could minimize wound tension and decrease the risk of keloid formation.

Fig. 7.2. Skin incision: deltopectoral approach

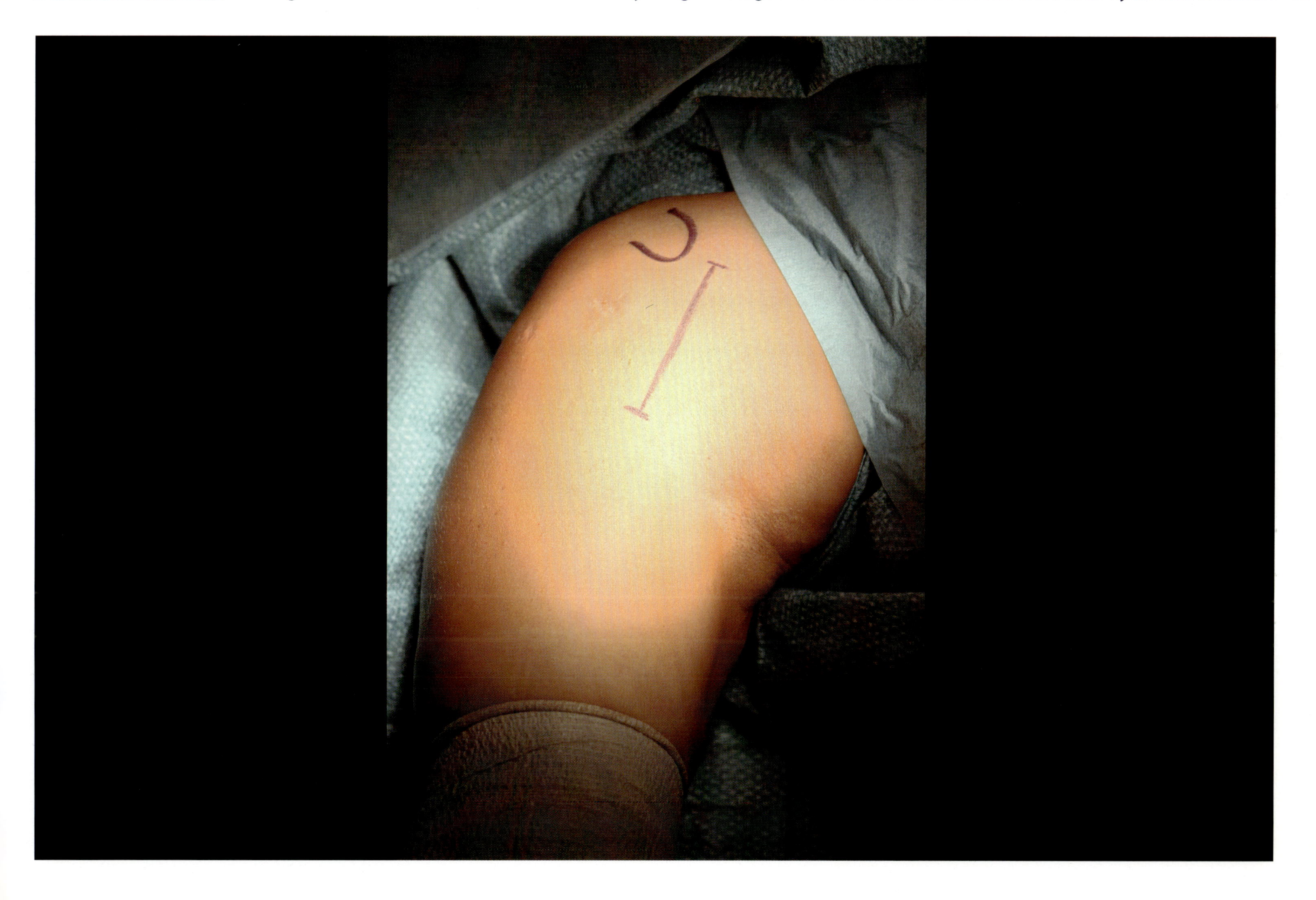

7.2.3 Deltopectoral Approach: Interval Opening

As seen in Fig. 7.3, the cephalic vein is identified proximally, preserved, and retracted laterally, ligating or cauterizing the medial branches from the deltoid muscle. Then the deltopectoral interval is opened. The clavipectoral fascia is divided just lateral to the conjoined tendon, preserving the coracoacromial ligament superiorly. Any overlaying subdeltoid bursa or adhesions from previous injury and surgery are excised, and the lesser tuberosity is identified. A self-retaining retractor is placed with one blade against the deltoid and the other against the coracoid muscles.

Tips and Tricks

Ligation or cauterization of the cephalic vein minimizes the risk of reoperation for postoperative bleeding.

Complication

The most common complication is hematoma formation, which usually resolves spontaneously, although some require aspiration(s) or drainage.

Fig. 7.3. Deltopectoral interval opening

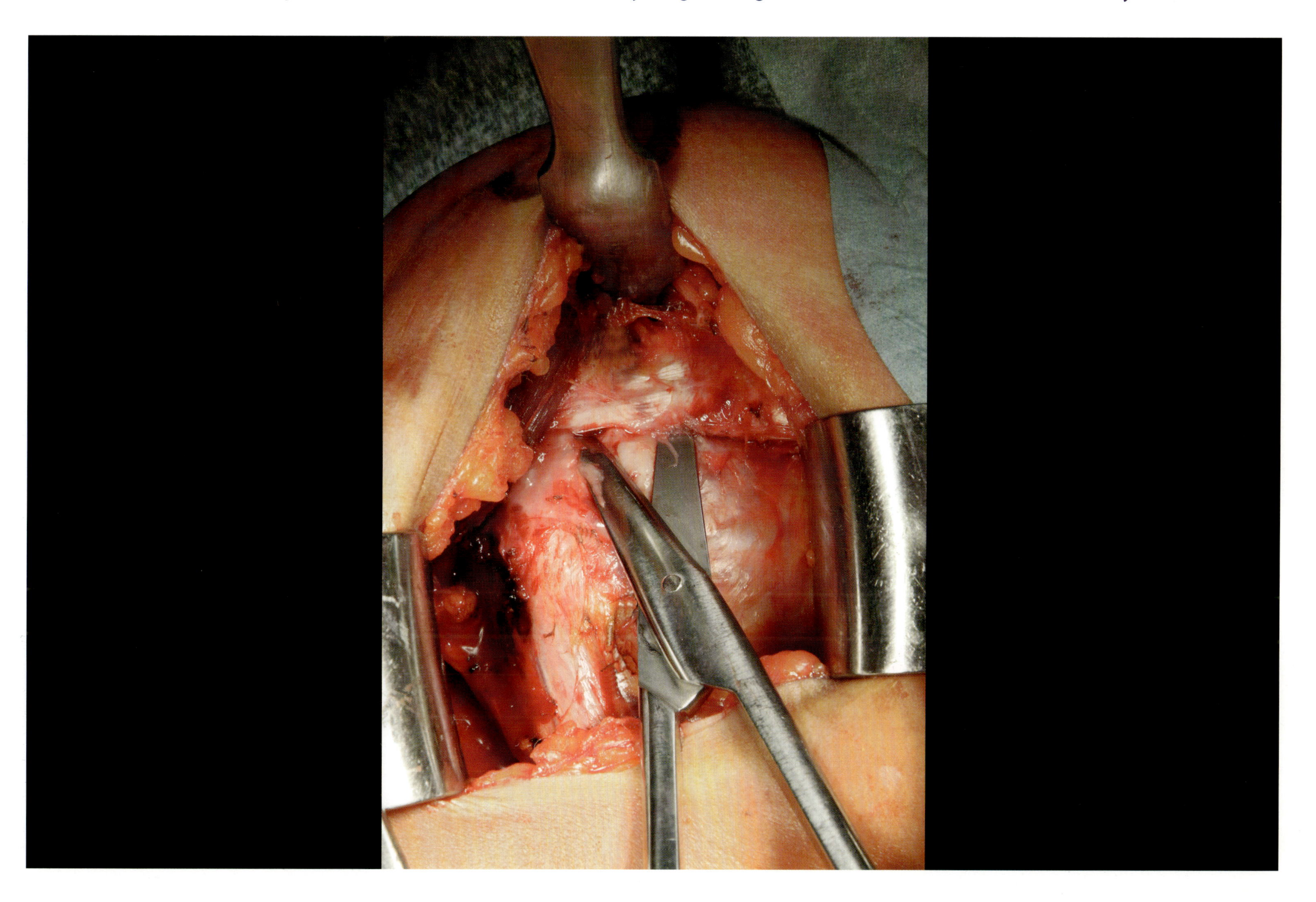

7.2.4 Subscapularis Tendon Split

Next, the arm is placed in a slight degree of external rotation to facilitate identification of the superior (rotator interval) and inferior (anterior humeral circumflex vessels) borders of the subscapularis tendon (Fig. 7.4). The rotator interval is easily identified 2–3 cm medial to tendon insertion on the humerus, and a large Kelly clamp is introduced just over the superior edge of the tendon. It is difficult to locate the rotator interval near the insertion, where the capsule and tendon blend. The subscapularis tendon is incised approximately at one third of its width from the inferior border.

Tips and Tricks
The subscapularis tendon and subjacent capsule are incised longitudinally, leaving sufficient distance from the lesser tuberosity to avoid damage of the biceps tendon reflection pulley. The axillary nerve is visualized and palpated and should be protected throughout this procedure. The axillary nerve can be located using the "tug" test: the index finger is swept beneath the coracoid process, over the subscapularis, and gently hooks the axillary nerve.

Complications
The most common complication is axillary nerve lesion.

Fig. 7.4. Subscapularis tendon split

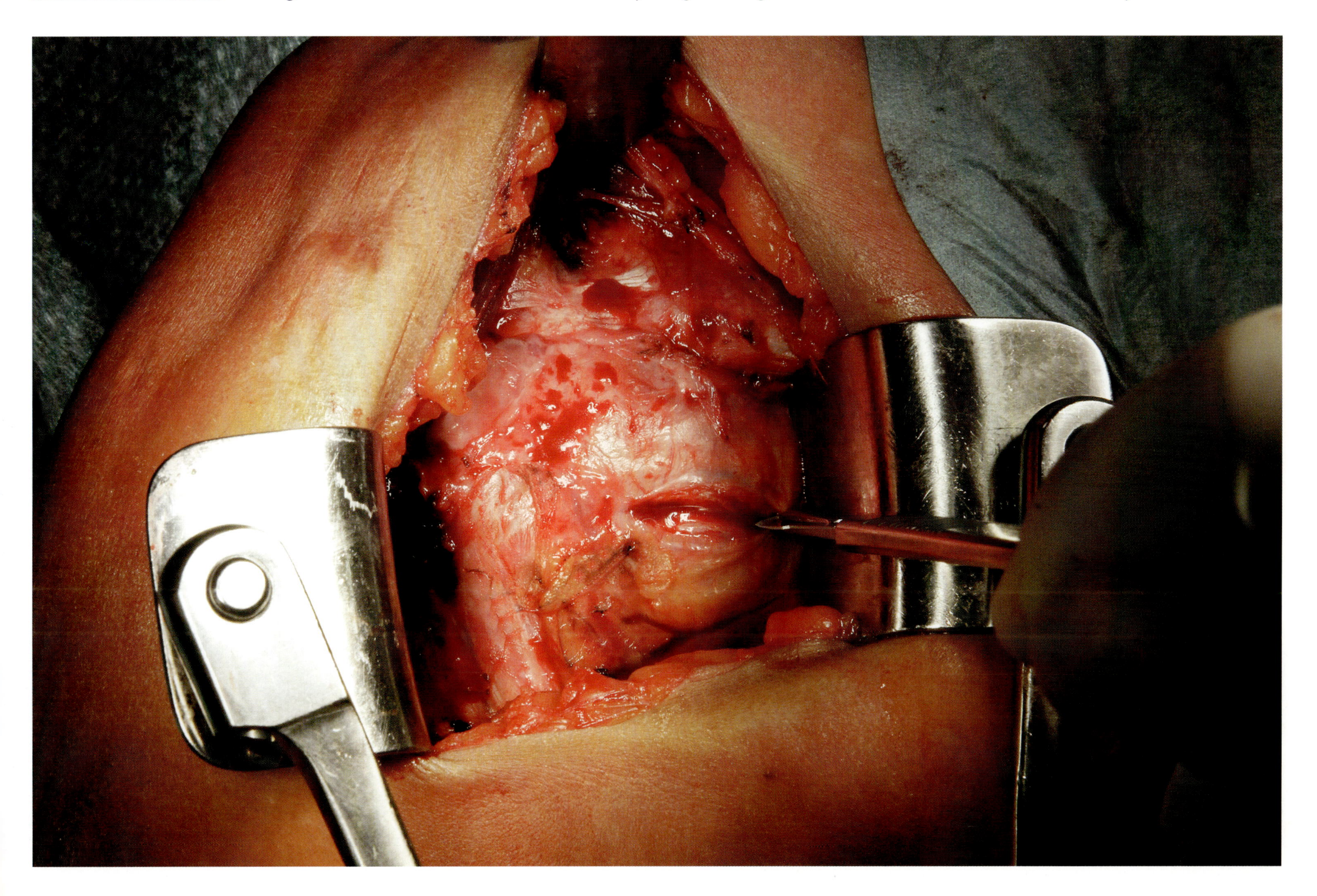

7.2.5 Capsulotomy

Using a sharp knife, the subscapularis tendon is separated from the underlying capsule; the plane of dissection is carried down to the anteroinferior glenoid neck. The capsule is incised horizontally in a "T" configuration between the middle and inferior glenohumeral ligaments, and traction sutures are placed in the superior and inferior borders of the capsule (Fig. 7.5).

Tips and Tricks

Previous scar tissue prevents separation between the subscapularis tendon and the capsule. The interval between subscapularis and capsule is more easily identified medially, and dissection may subsequently be carried out with a small sponge.

Complications

As in the previous step, the most frequent complication is axillary nerve lesion.

Fig. 7.5. Horizontal capsulotomy

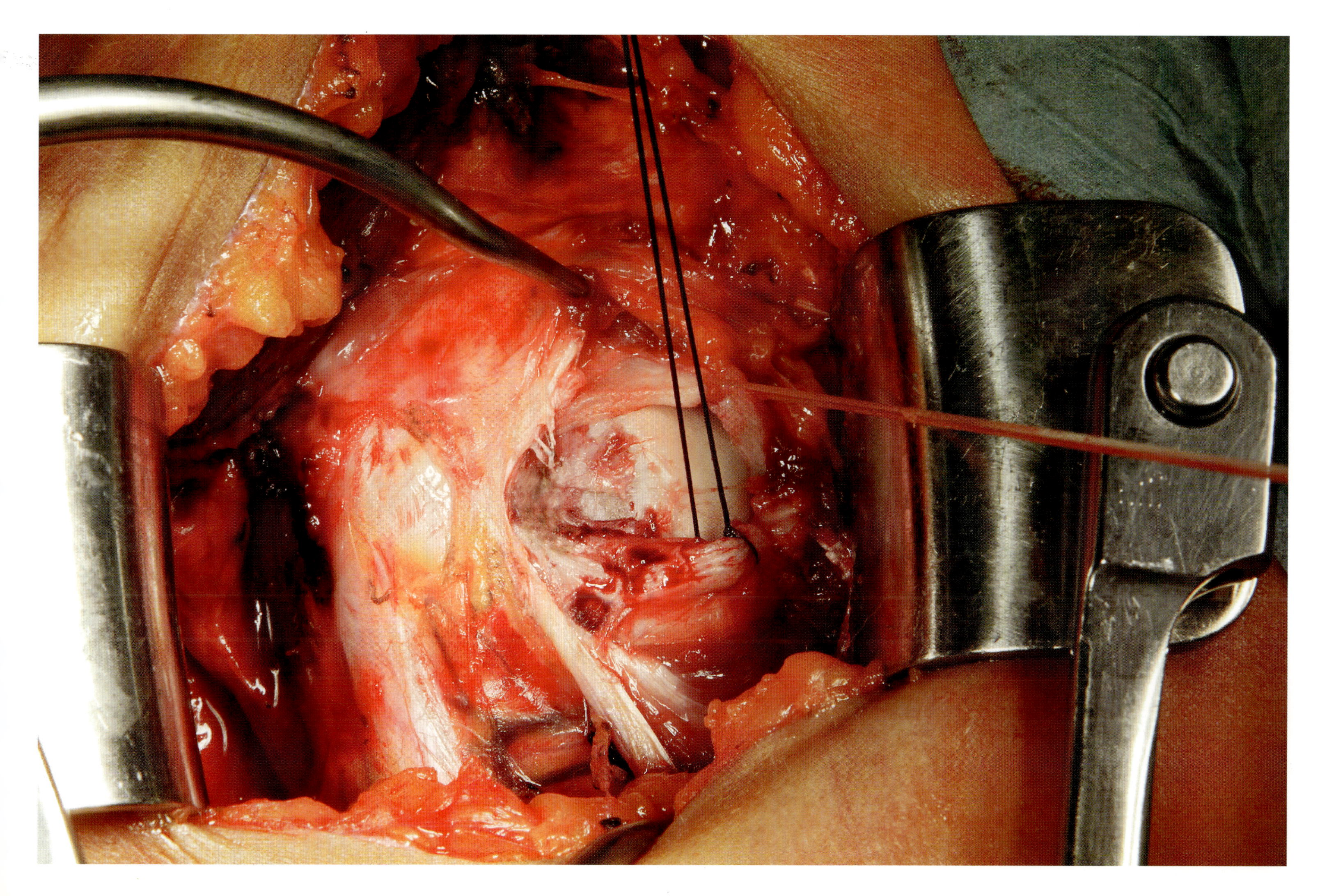

7.2.6 Exposing the Glenoid (1)

A Fukuda ring retractor is placed to subluxate the humeral head posteriorly, and a spiked retractor is placed on the anterior glenoid neck to retract the capsule medially to inspect the joint (Fig. 7.6).

Tips and Tricks

Obtaining adequate glenoid exposure may be the most difficult part of the entire operation. One of the most important requirements for adequate glenoid exposure is muscular paralysis. If an interscalene block has been used, this alone can produce excellent muscular relaxation.

Complications

Nerve dysfunction related to traction neurapraxia.

Fig. 7.6. Exposing the glenoid: placement of Fukuda ring retractor and spiked retractor

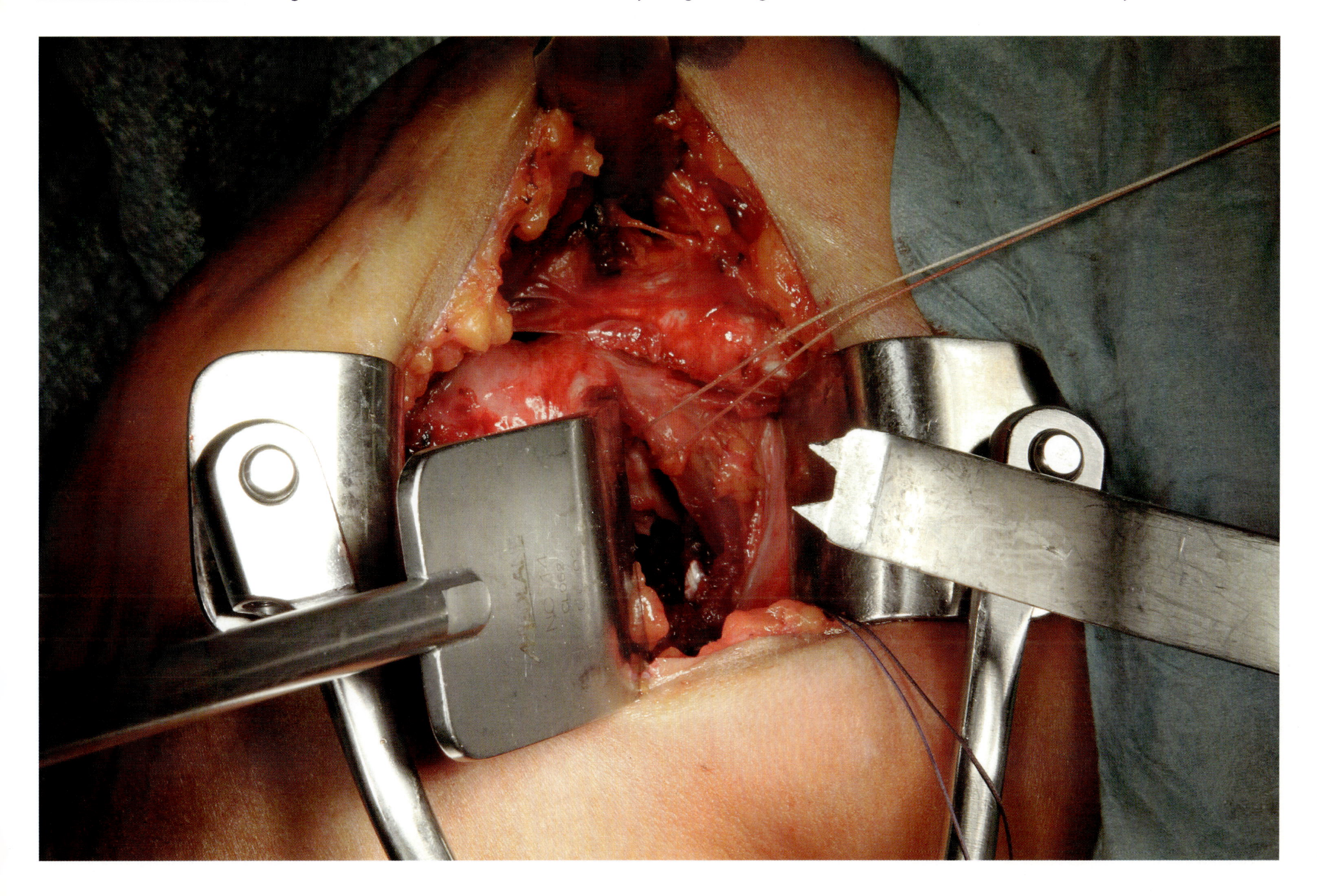

7.2.7 Exposing the Glenoid (2)

The choice of retractors and their placement are key in attaining good glenoid exposure. To improve visualization of the glenoid neck, the capsule must be displaced superiorly with a Steinman rod and inferiorly with a small Hohmann retractor (the latter is not routinely necessary) (Fig. 7.7).

Tips and Tricks

Periarticular soft tissue contracture can limit glenoid exposure, so additional anteroinferior capsular release may be required, with the axillary nerve retracted using a small Hohmann retractor.

Complications

As in the previous step, the most frequent complication is nerve dysfunction related to traction neurapraxia.

Fig. 7.7. Exposing the glenoid: placement of Steinman rod and Hohmann retractor

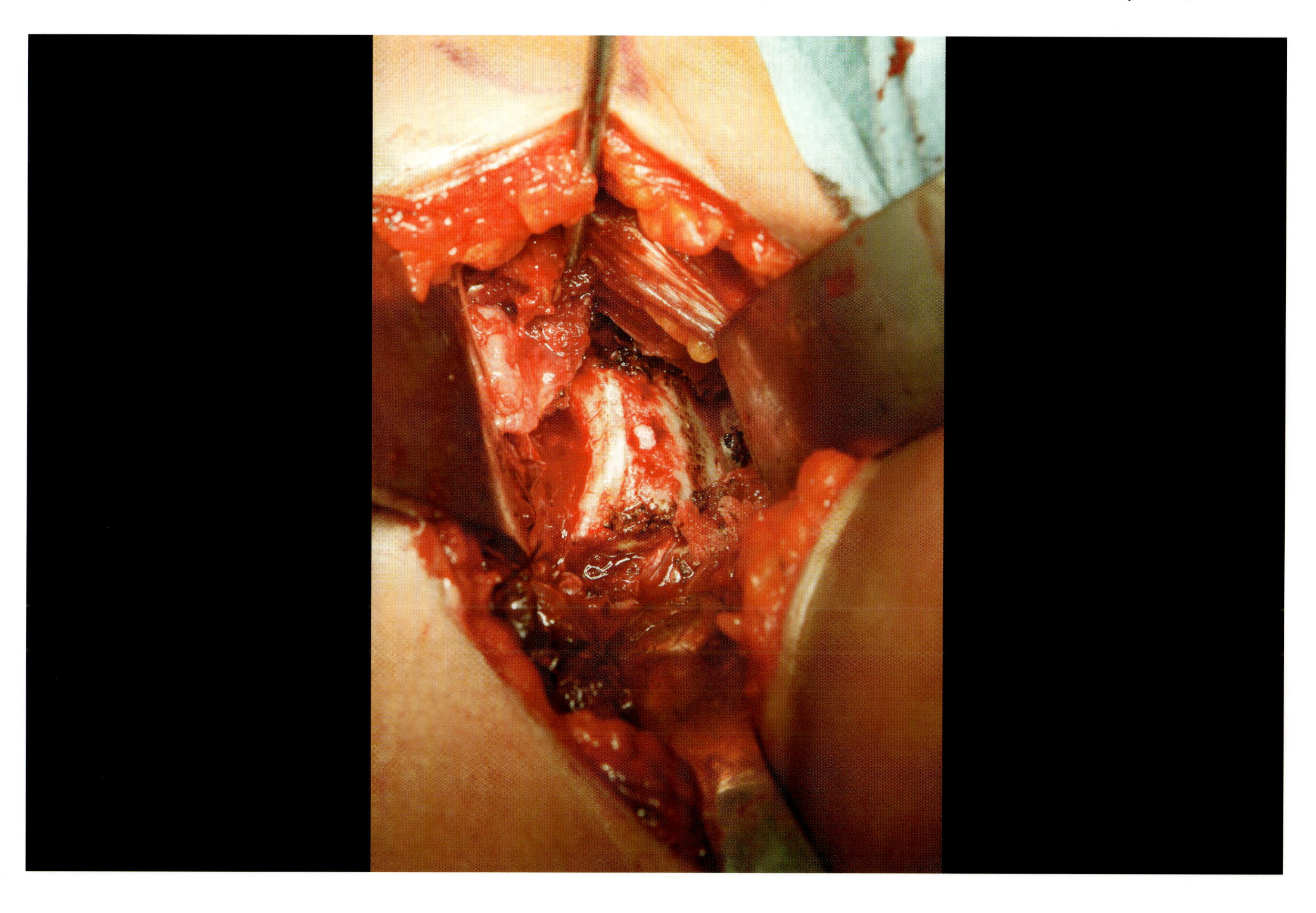

7.2.8 Glenoid Defect Measurement

The anteroinferior glenoid neck is identified by removing all scar tissue, and the bone defect is measured. The defect site is then prepared with a high-speed olive-shaped burr to obtain a smooth surface (Fig. 7.8).

Tips and Tricks

The length of the osseous defect is measured and compared with the width of the maximum glenoid anteroposterior radius. The measured defect length is the basis for the size of the iliac-crest bone graft to be harvested.

Complications

Insufficient bone-graft size. To avoid this complication, size of the glenoid osseous defect filled is measured before tricortical graft is harvested.

Fig. 7.8. Glenoid-defect measurement

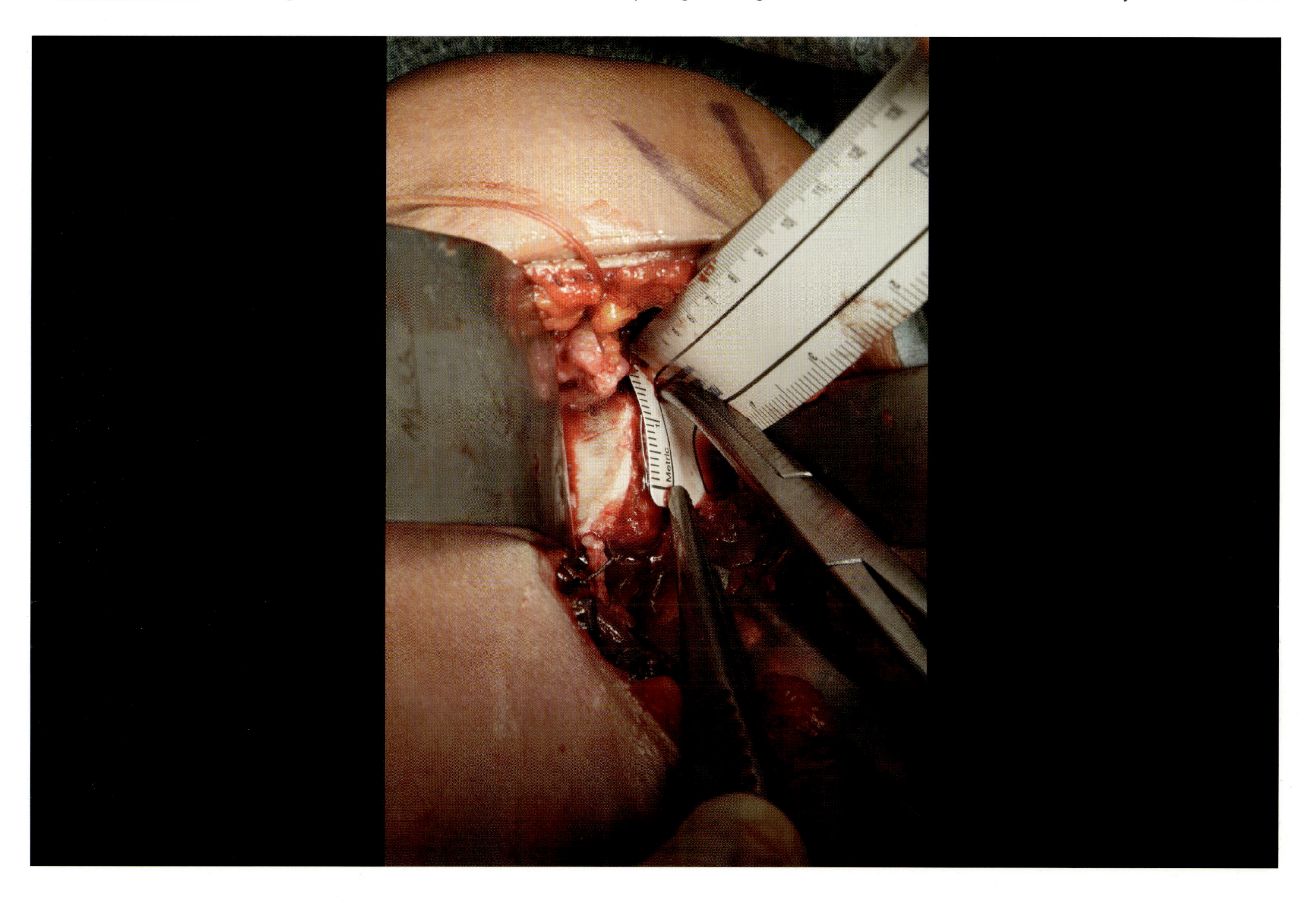
Metric

7.2.9 Autologous Anterior Iliac-crest Bone Graft: Incision

Attention is then directed to the ipsilateral anterior iliac crest for the harvest. A skin incision is made along the crest line, just behind the anterior superior iliac spine. The lateral femoral cutaneous nerve crosses the medial aspect of the anterior superior iliac spine (ASIS) at a distance between 15 and 50 mm of the ASIS, so injury of this nerve is unlikely if the incision remains 2 cm lateral to the ASIS. To take a tricortical graft involving the full thickness of the iliac wing, the aponeurosis must be incised along the apex of the iliac crest. Both internal and external iliac fossae are then exposed by reflecting superiorly the iliacus, in continuity with the abdominal muscles, and the glutei inferiorly (Fig. 7.9).

Tips and Tricks

Skin incision length is variable based on graft size needed, but it can be retracted as a mobile window with the use of small retractors. We recommend placing the incision off the most prominent aspect of the iliac crest to minimize postoperative scar sensitivity and irritation from clothing, such as waistbands and belts.

Complications

Injury to the lateral femoral cutaneous nerve is the most common complication. The two major injury mechanisms are: (1) direct damage or electrocauterization of the nerve, and (2) neurapraxia from excessive tension during retraction of the iliac muscles while exposing the inner table of the ilium.

Fig. 7.9. Anterior iliac-crest bone graft: skin incision

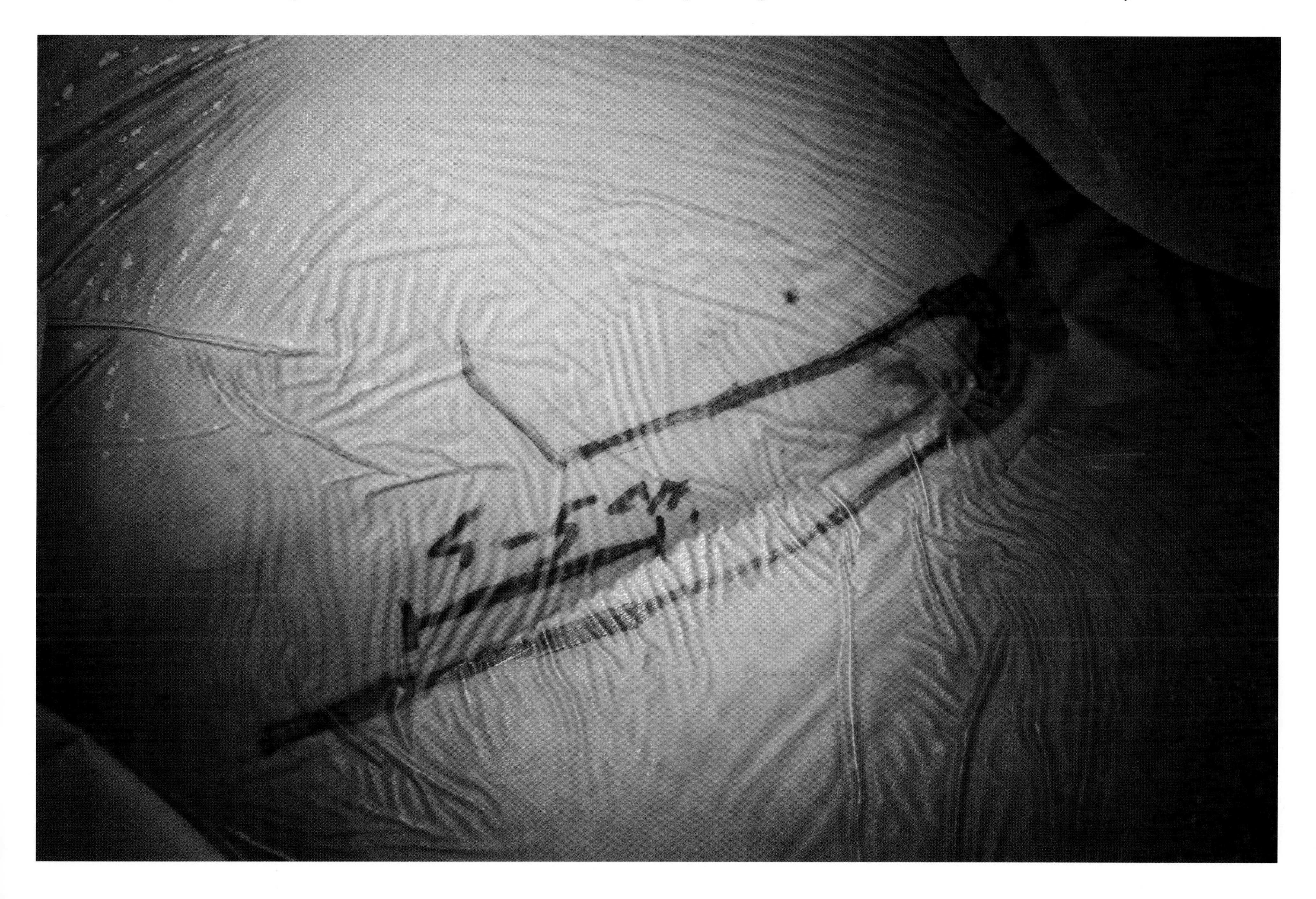
4-5 cm.

7.2.10 Anterior Iliac-crest Bone Graft Harvest

As shown in Fig. 7.10, a structural graft is harvested from the middle section of the iliac crest to obtain a mildly curved surface that precisely fits the area of the glenoid defect. The size of the bone graft is determined by the size of the recipient defect. This graft usually measures approximately 8-mm thick, 1-cm deep, and 3-cm wide. Before removing the tricortical graft, the area is outlined with an indelible pencil. The graft may then be removed more easily with a power saw (an oscillating saw or an air-powered cutting drill). This technique is also less traumatic than when an osteotome and hammer are used. After removing the graft, the periosteum and muscular origins are accurately apposed and held with strong, interrupted sutures. Bleeding from the ilium is sometimes profuse; gentle wound suction for 24–48 h could be quite satisfactory for managing this wound.

Tips and Tricks

The inner and outer tables of the anterior ilium are exposed by elevating the fascia subperiosteally, with electrocautery to avoid bleeding and hematoma formation.

Complications

Avulsion fracture of the anterior superior iliac spine can occur following anterior bone-graft harvest. Iliac fracture is most effectively avoided through judicious limitation of bone-graft harvest a minimum of 3 cm lateral to the anterior superior iliac spine.

Fig. 7.10. Anterior iliac-crest bone-graft harvest from the middle part of the crest

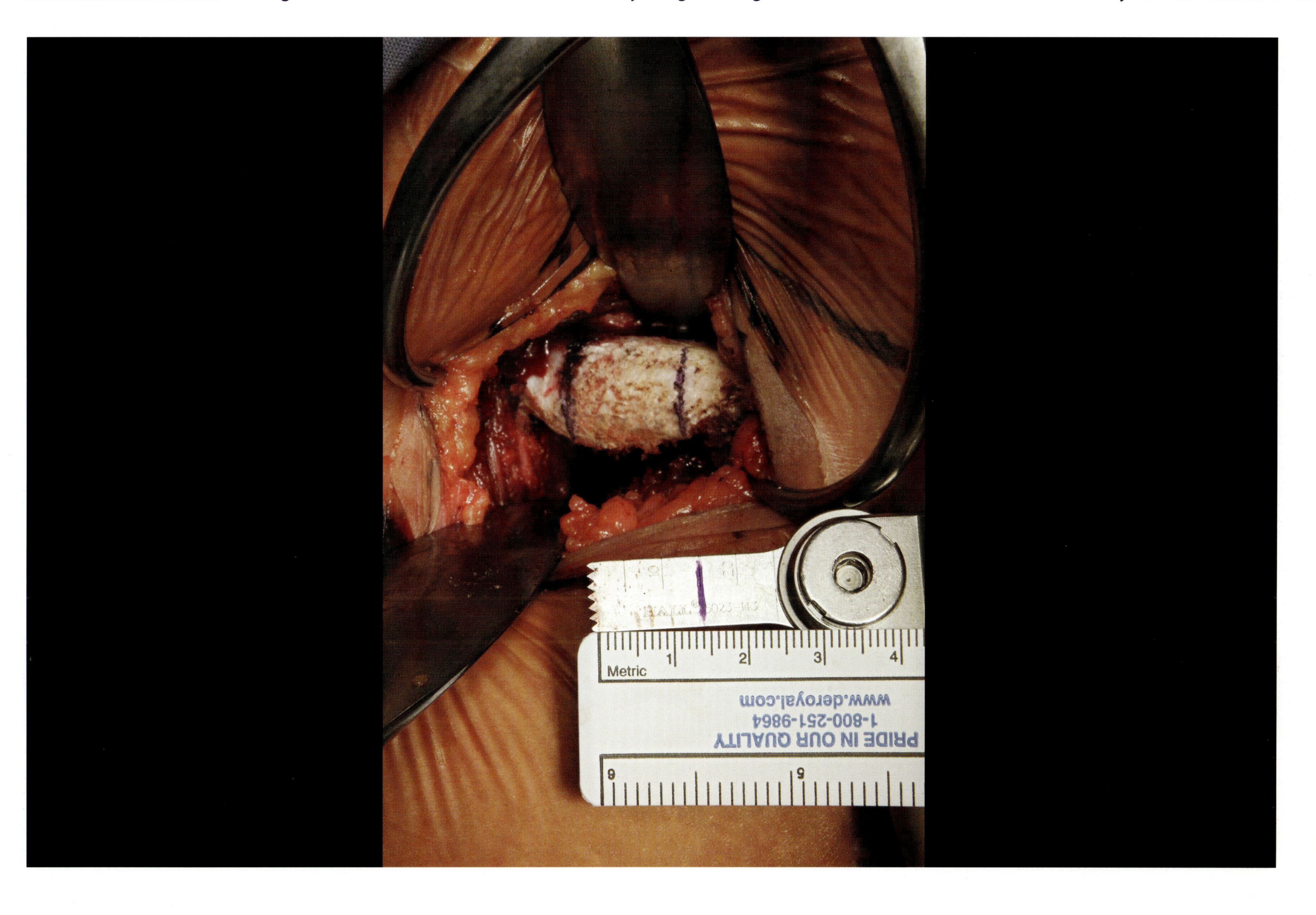
Metric
www.deroyal.com
1-800-251-9864
PRIDE IN OUR QUALITY

7.2.11 Placement and Fixation of the Anterior Iliac-crest Bone Graft

The graft is contoured using a small saw and burr so that the graft fits onto the anterior glenoid in a fashion that adds width and depth to the glenoid surface. The graft is placed beneath the equator and level with the edge of the anterior glenoid, with the inner cortical concave table anteriorly. The bone-graft surface should be flush with the native articular surface. The graft is temporary fixed with 2 (or 3) Kirschner wires and then secured to the glenoid with two or three self-tapping screws using a standard technique. The screws must be bicortical (Fig. 7.11).

Tips and Tricks

The angle between graft and scapular neck is inclined to add correct joint concavity. The wires must be oriented medially and parallel to the joint surface so that the screw heads set medially, as far away from the humeral articular surface as possible.

Complications

Angulating the graft placement too far may result in humeral-head impingement and articular erosion. Another possible complication is bone-graft fracture, which can be avoided by using the so-called "two-fingers" technique when tightening screws.

Fig. 7.11. Placement and fixation of anterior iliac-crest bone graft

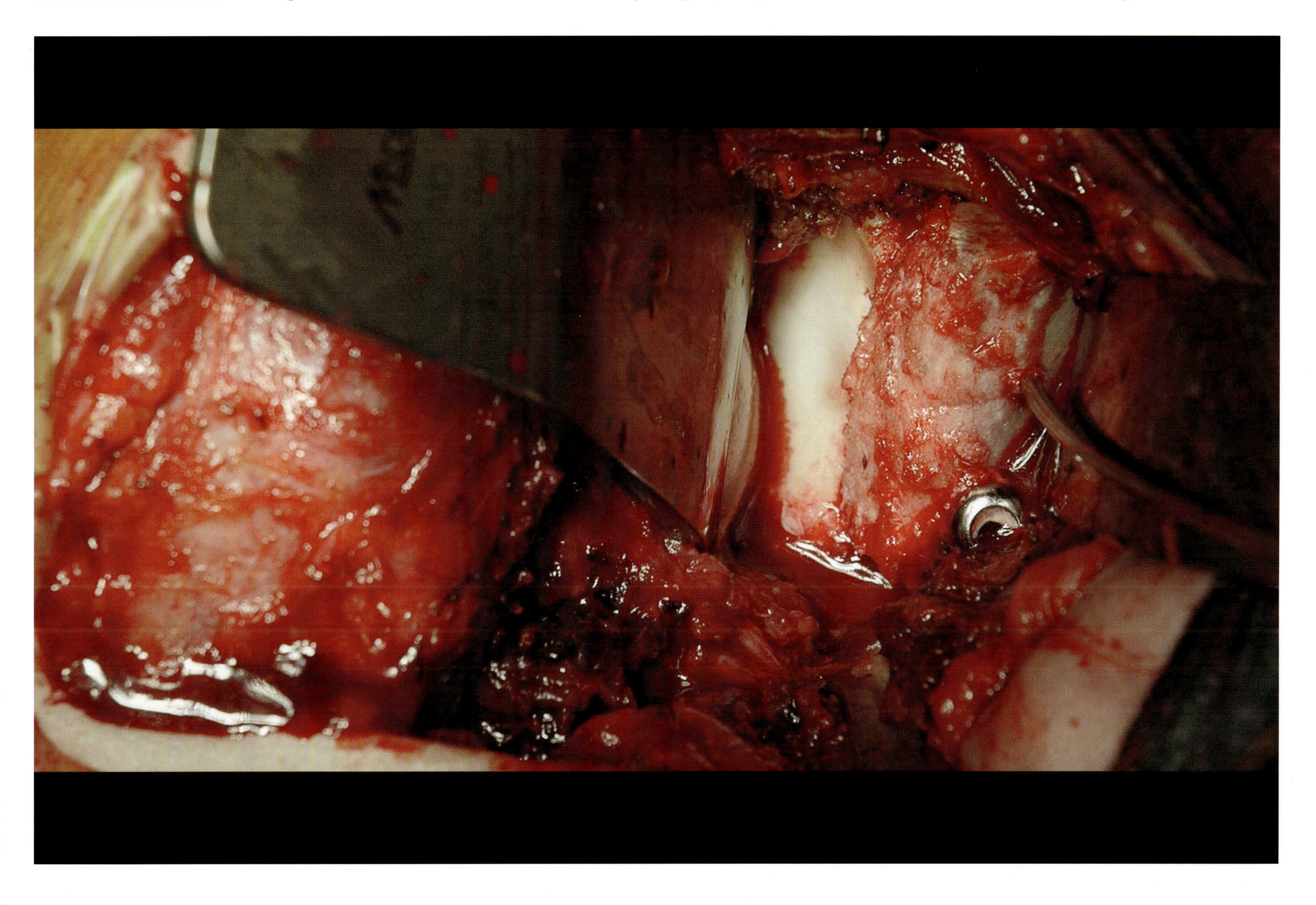

7.2.12 Remodeling the Anterior Iliac-crest Bone Graft

Once the graft is secured, the interface between graft and glenoid surface is visualized and palpated to confirm a smooth transition and glenoid depth restoration (concavity). If necessary, the graft can be contoured further to remove any prominence or extension beyond the curvature of the glenoid articular surface. The humeral retractor is then removed, and humeral-head positioning on the newly reconstructed glenoid is assessed by rotating the arm (Fig. 7.12).

Tips and Tricks
When ideally positioned, the graft should not be touched by the humeral head before 20–30° of external rotation to avoid early graft contact.

Complications
Bone graft overhang may lead to arthrosis.

Fig. 7.12. Remodeling anterior iliac-crest bone graft

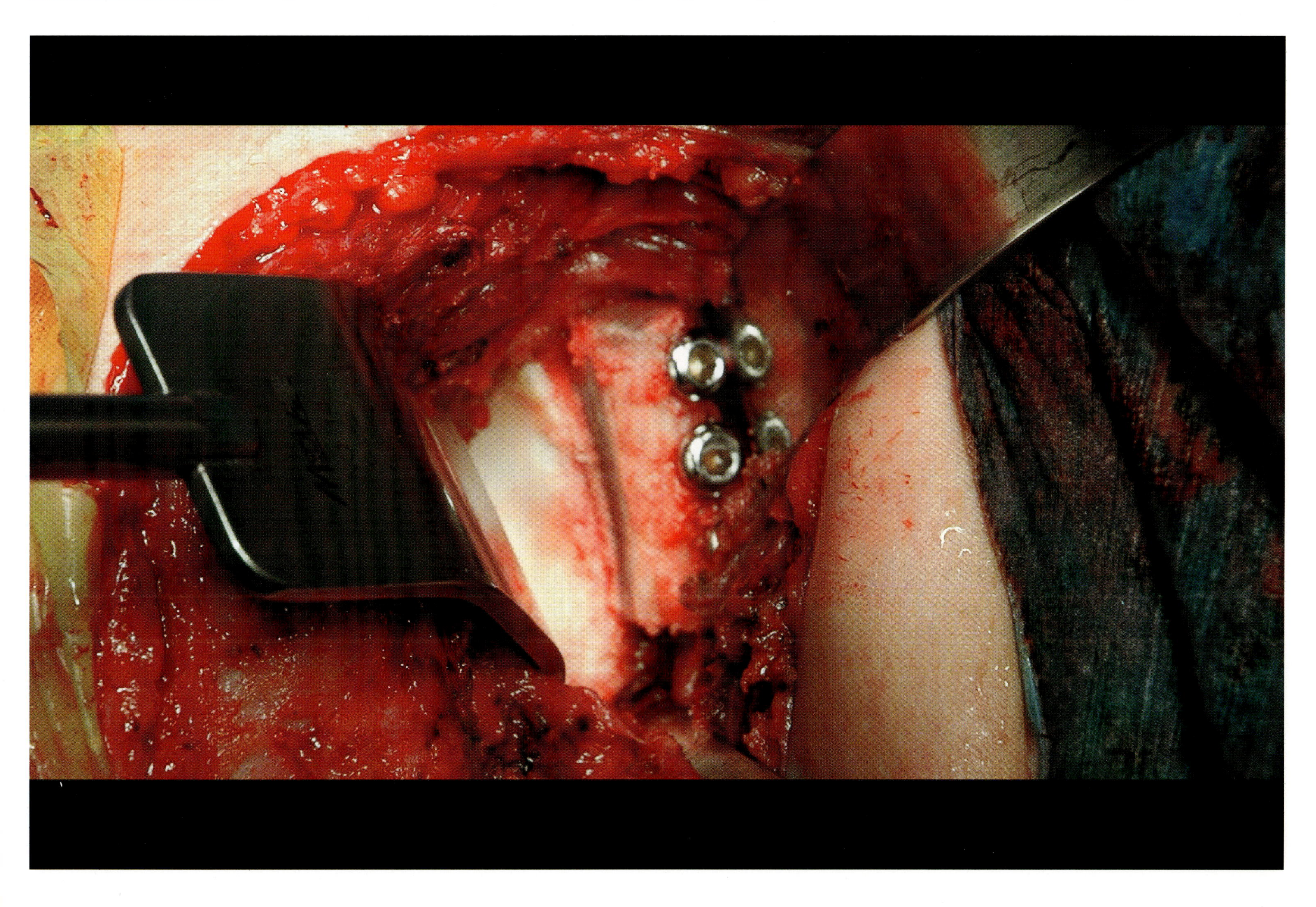

7.2.13 Capsule Repair and Closure

Soft tissue closure requires secure repair of the anterior capsular complex and routine closure of the subscapularis tendon split (Fig. 7.13). The "T" incision of the capsule allows shifting the inferior capsular flap in the superior direction to eliminate the redundant inferior pouch. Deltopectoral interval, subcutaneous tissues, and skin can be routinely closed with interrupted sutures over a suction drainage tube. Dry, sterile dressings are applied, and the patient is returned to the recovery room with the arm in a sling.

Tips and Tricks

The capsule is repaired with the arm in approximately 30° of external rotation and 30° of abduction.

Complications

Postoperatively, patients will experience some stiffness and should be counseled to expect some limitation of external rotation. The goal is to achieve a stable joint with no more than 20° loss of external rotation to limit the risk of capsulorrhaphy arthropathy.

7.3 Postoperative Treatment

Postoperatively, immobilizing abduction (15°) shoulder sling supports the shoulder for the first 6 weeks. The patient removes the arm from the sling several times a day to perform pendulum exercises. Rehabilitation is initiated on the third postoperative week and progresses through three phases: Phase I – passive- and active-assisted range of motion in elevation and external rotation within safe limits as defined by intraoperative testing. The goals during this phase focus on edema control and a gentle increase in joint mobility to avoid stiffness and scarring. Phase II – from 6 to 12 weeks, includes active and active-assisted range of motion and initiation of gentle stretching with care not to stress the repair. The goals during this phase focus on improving functional active motion and coordinating scapular-humeral rhythm. Patients are encouraged to begin light activities of daily living as tolerated. Phase III – beginning at 12 weeks, this phase involves gradual muscle strengthening. The goals are aimed at maximizing shoulder functional capacity in activities of daily living in addition to improving strength and endurance. Return to work is determined on an individual basis but is generally allowed between 4 and 6 months postoperatively.

Fig. 7.13. Capsule repair

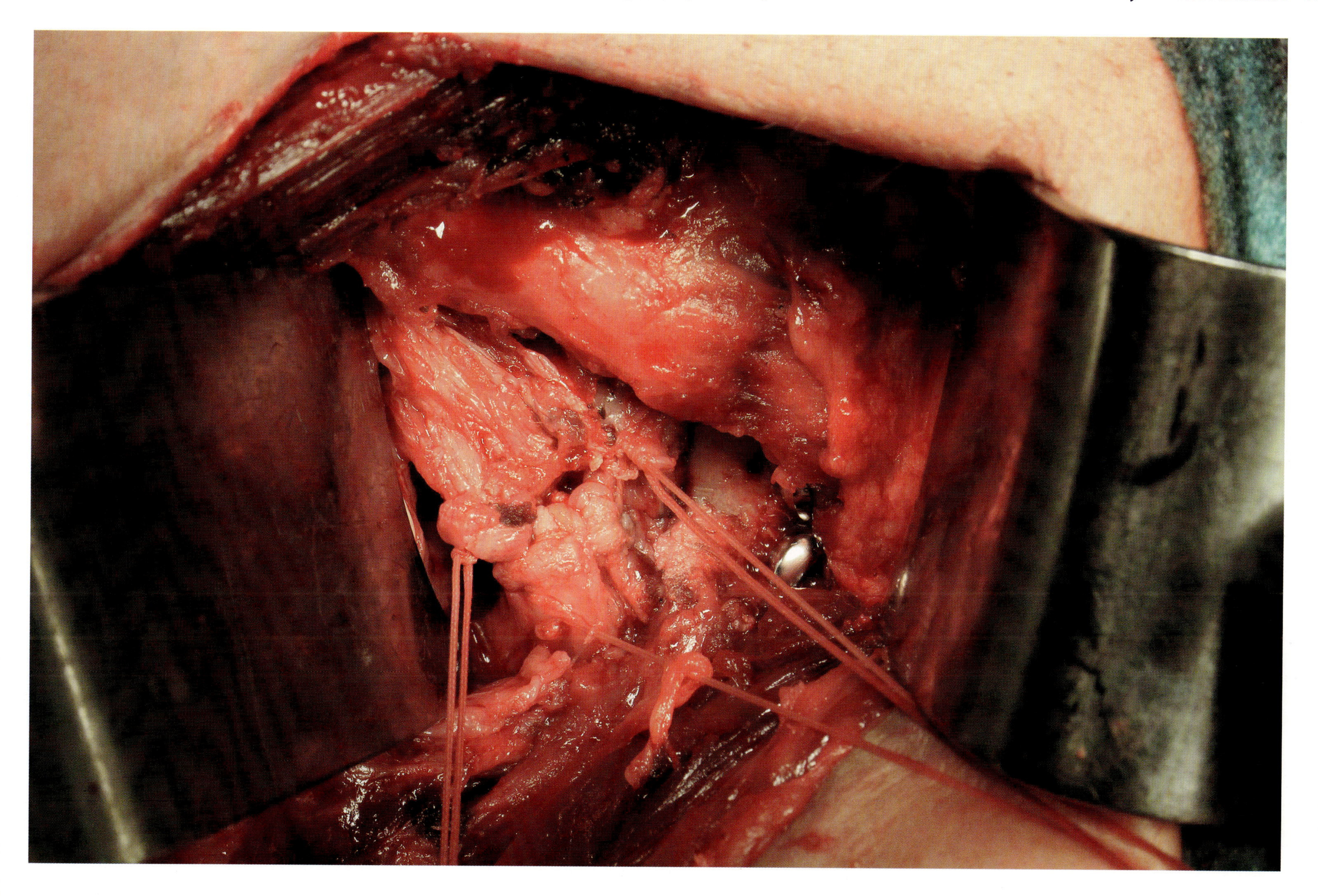

7.4 Critical Concepts

7.4.1 Indications

- Recurrent anteroinferior glenohumeral instability with glenoid bone loss >30%;
- failure of other types of bone grafting for anterior stabilization, such as a Bristow or a Latarjet.

7.4.2 Contraindications

- Active infection in the operative area;
- high risk of poor patient compliance, especially due to substance abuse (drugs and/or alcohol);
- elderly patient with a rotator-cuff deficiency;
- glenohumeral arthropathy;
- very large humeral head defect (relative contraindication), although glenoid grafting still may be useful in conjunction with a humeral hemiarthroplasty in selected circumstances.

7.4.3 Pitfalls

The main pitfall, as with any shoulder articular surgical procedure, is related to glenoid exposure and preparation. Failure to achieve proper exposure prevents the consistent glenoid preparation required for successful graft placement and fixation. We believe that adequate exposure is greatly facilitated by proper patient positioning and appropriate soft tissue release. When the optimal exposure is achieved, another pitfall to avoid is inappropriate bone-graft placement, which must be flush with the glenoid surface. This technique is applicable in any situation requiring glenoid augmentation and is particularly useful in cases of deficient glenoid bone stock, such as is found in recurrent shoulder instability.

7.4.4 Authors' Update

There are no absolute indications for this procedure. We consider anterior glenoid tricortical iliac-crest bone grafting only for informed patients who the surgeon believes are acceptable surgical candidates, specifically in whom a previous bone graft has failed and soft tissue repair is not likely to succeed.

References

1. Beran MC, Donaldson CT, Bishop JY (2010) Treatment of chronic glenoid defects in the setting of recurrent anterior shoulder instability: a systematic review. J Shoulder Elbow Surg 19:769-780
2. Lynch JR, Clinton JM, Dewing CB et al (2009) Treatment of osseous defects associated with anterior shoulder instability. J Shoulder Elbow Surg 18:317-328
3. Burkhart SS, De Beer JF (2000) Traumatic glenohumeral bone defects and their relationship to failure of arthroscopic Bankart repairs: significance of the inverted-pear glenoid and the humeral engaging Hill-Sachs lesion. Arthroscopy 16:677-694
4. Itoi E, Lee SB, Berglund LJ et al (2000) The effect of a glenoid defect on anteroinferior stability of the shoulder after Bankart repair: a cadaveric study. J Bone Joint Surg Am 82:35-46
5. Yamamoto N, Muraki T, Sperling JW et al (2010) Stabilizing mechanism in bone-grafting of a large glenoid defect. J Bone Joint Surg Am 92:2059-2066
6. Baudi P, Righi P, Bolognesi D et al (2005) How to identify and calculate glenoid bone deficit. Chir Organi Mov 90:145-152
7. Wellmann M, Petersen W, Zantop T et al (2009) Open shoulder repair of osseous glenoid defects: biomechanical effectiveness of the Latarjet procedure versus a contoured structural bone graft. Am J Sports Med 37:87-94
8. Warner JJ, Gill TJ, O'hollerhan JD et al (2006) Anatomical glenoid reconstruction for recurrent anterior glenohumeral instability with glenoid deficiency using an autogenous tricortical iliac crest bone graft. Am J Sports Med 34:205-212

9. Ghodadra N, Gupta A, Romeo AA et al (2010) Normalization of glenohumeral articular contact pressures after Latarjet or iliac crest bone-grafting. J Bone Joint Surg Am 92:1478-1489
10. Montgomery WH Jr, Wahl M, Hettrich C et al (2005) Anteroinferior bone-grafting can restore stability in osseous glenoid defects. J Bone Joint Surg Am 87:1972-1977
11. Matsen FA III, Chebli C, Lippit SB (2007) Open anterior shoulder repair with glenoid bone loss. In: Zuckerman JD (ed) Advanced reconstruction shoulder. American Academy of Orthopaedic Surgeons, Rosemont, pp 77-84
12. Eden R (1918) Zur Operations der habituellen Schulterluxation unter Mitteilung eines neuen Verfahrens bei Abriss am inneren Pfannenrande. Deutsch Ztschr Chir 144:268-280
13. Hybbinette S (1932) De la transplantation d'un fragment osseux pour remedier aux luxations recidivantes de l'epaule; constatations et resultats operatoires. Acta Chir Scand 71:411-445
14. Rahme H, Wikblad L, Nowak J et al (2003) Long-term clinical and radiologic results after Eden-Hybbinette operation for anterior instability of the shoulder. J Shoulder Elbow Surg 12:15-19
15. Brox JI, Finnanger AM, Merckoll E et al (2003) Satisfactory long-term results after Eden-Hybbinette-Alvik operation for recurrent anterior dislocation of the shoulder: 6-20 years' follow-up of 52 patients. Acta Orthop Scand 74:180-185
16. Lindholm TS (1974) Results of treatment for anterior recurrent dislocation of the shoulder joint with the Eden-Hybbinette operation. Acta Orthop Scand 45:508-517
17. Rachbauer F, Ogon M, Wimmer C et al (2000) Glenohumeral osteoarthrosis after the Eden-Hybbinette procedure. Clin Orthop Relat Res 373:135-140

Chapter 8 – Focal Resurfacing of Humeral-head Defects

Pradeep Kodali, Anthony Miniaci

8.1 Introduction

Traumatic shoulder instability is extremely common in athletes. It is usually due to abnormal abduction, external rotation, and extension force on the shoulder, causing it to exceed normal limits of glenohumeral motion and resulting in anterior dislocation. A characteristic anteroinferior capsulolabral injury occurs and has been deemed the essential lesion in anterior shoulder instability [1–3]. A posterosuperior humeral-head defect (Hill-Sachs lesion) is noted in 93% of cases [4]. This bone defect, if large enough, may contribute to failed soft tissue stabilization that occurs in 8–18% of patients [4–6]. Large defects lead to an articular arc mismatch that, at lesser degrees of external rotation, will engage with the anteroinferior glenoid, causing instability [7]. Treatment typically entails a combined procedure to address the soft tissue injury and bone defect. For large Hill-Sachs lesions, surgical options include nonanatomic techniques, such as the remplissage procedure [4, 8], or anatomic techniques. Purchase et al. [8] used an arthroscopic remplissage technique and had only a 7% chance of recurrent instability. Anatomic techniques include either matched humeral-head allograft or resurfacing arthroplasty with HemiCAP© (Arthrosurface, Franklin, MA, USA) [9]. Allograft transplantation for Hill-Sachs lesions has been described and yields good outcomes in most case reports [10–12]. One series of 18 patients with humeral-head defects >25% of the humeral-head diameter and treated with structural allografts showed no evidence of recurrent instability 2 years after surgery [13]. Recently, due to the difficulty of obtaining matched allografts, patients have lent toward electing a resurfacing procedure, which have yielded positive early results (unpublished data). Our preference is anatomic reconstruction, which is the focus of this chapter.

8.2 Indication/Algorithm

Our indication for treating humeral-head defects relies largely on physical examination in combination with imaging studies identifying a large humeral-head defect. In our experience, apprehension with the arm at 45° of abduction and 45° of external rotation indicates a significant bony injury, contributing to instability in a functional range of motion. If there is no apprehension with this maneuver, then a soft tissue procedure will likely suffice. Preoperative workup includes plain radiographs [anteroposterior (AP), true AP, axillary, scapular Y], computed tomography (CT) scan, and a magnetic resonance imaging (MRI) study. Although there are various radiographic techniques to quantify the size of the humeral-head defect [14–16], there is no universally accepted method or criterion that dictates treatment. Recently, Sekiya et al. [17], in a biomechanical study, showed that defects as small 12.5% of the humeral head affect stability and may benefit from allograft transplantation [17]. Kaar et al. [18], in another biomechanical study, showed that defects that are five eighths of the radius of the humeral head affect stability. We use the various imaging studies to determine the extent of soft tissue injury and confirm the presence of a large humeral-head or glenoid-rim defect. A combination of a large humeral-head defect with positive physical exam findings necessitates addressing the bony injury, thus requiring an open procedure.

8.3 Technique: Humeral-head Resurfacing with Artificial Implant

We position the patient in a modified beach-chair position with the operative extremity free in order to allow adequate extension and external rotation of the arm. The deltopectoral approach is used even for posterior humeral-head defects, because with appropriate arm positioning and adequate capsular release, the defect is clearly visualized. In addition, the soft tissue injury can be addressed at the same time, eliminating the need for a separate incision. An 8- to 10-cm incision is made along the deltopectoral groove lateral to the coracoid process (Fig. 8.1). The incision can be extended proximally to

Fig. 8.1. Incision for the deltopectoral approach

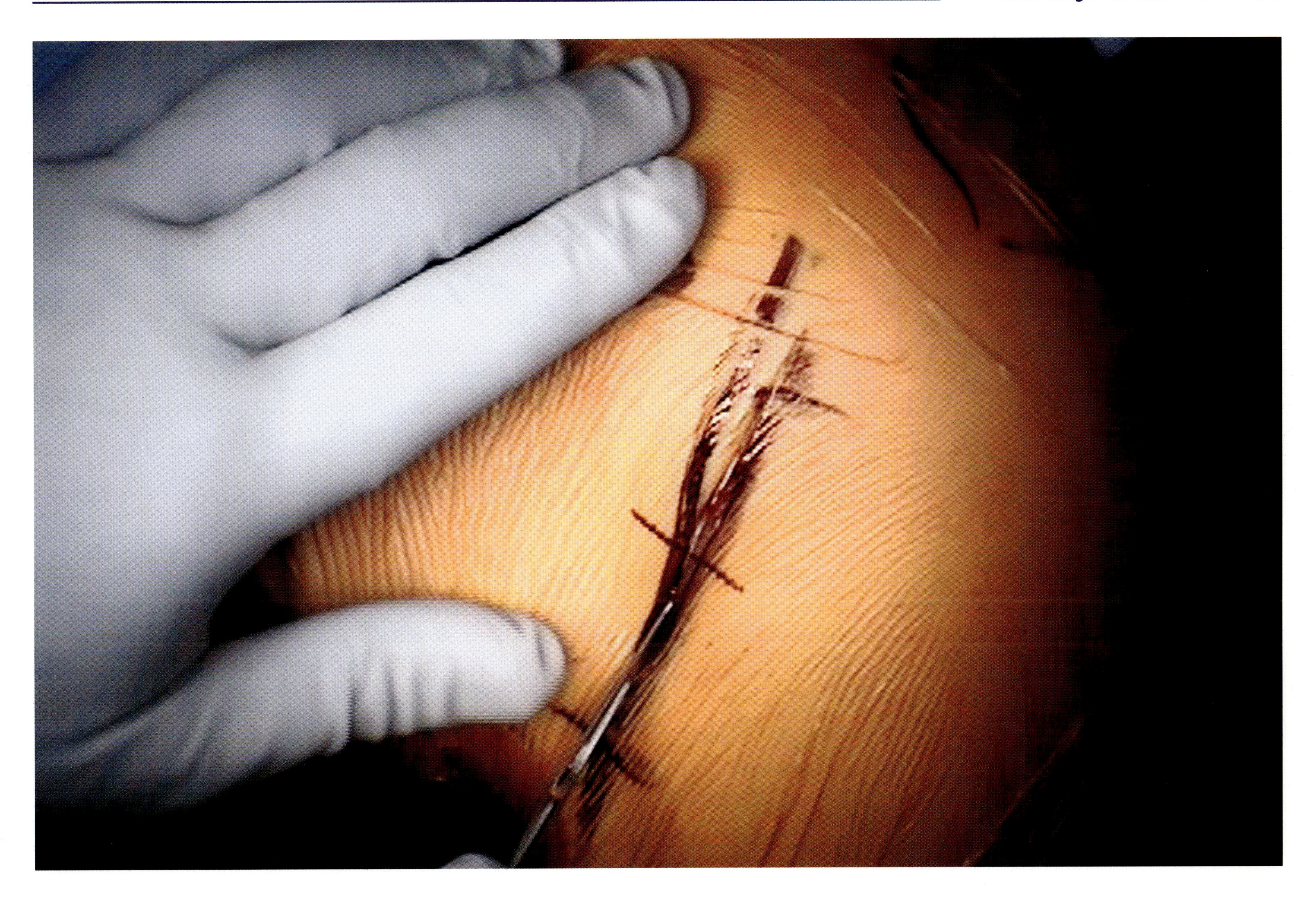

the clavicle and distally along the medial border of the deltoid as far as needed. The cephalic vein is identified, and the interval is developed medial to the vein. It is important to visualize insertion of pectoralis major, and partial release of this may facilitate exposure. After dissection through the clavipectoral fascia, the subscapularis is identified (Fig. 8.2). A longitudinal incision is made through the subscapularis and capsule ensuring 1 cm of subscapularis tendon is left on the humeral side, facilitating later repair. The capsule is now separated from the subscapularis and tagged with a suture. The arm is positioned in extension and external rotation to place tension on the inferior capsule, and the capsule is released from the humerus using a cautery device. Adequate capsular release is integral to obtaining sufficient exposure of the Hill-Sachs lesion (Fig. 8.3). A humeral-head retractor is used to inspect the glenoid for labral pathology. If the classic Bankart lesion is seen, it is repaired with suture anchors. The sutures are passed through the labrum but are not tied until the conclusion of the resurfacing procedure. At this point, instrumentation for the HemiCAP resurfacing system is used. Appropriately sized

Fig. 8.2. Subscapularis is visualized after dissection through the interval

Fig. 8.3. Hill-Sachs lesion is exposed (*arrows*)

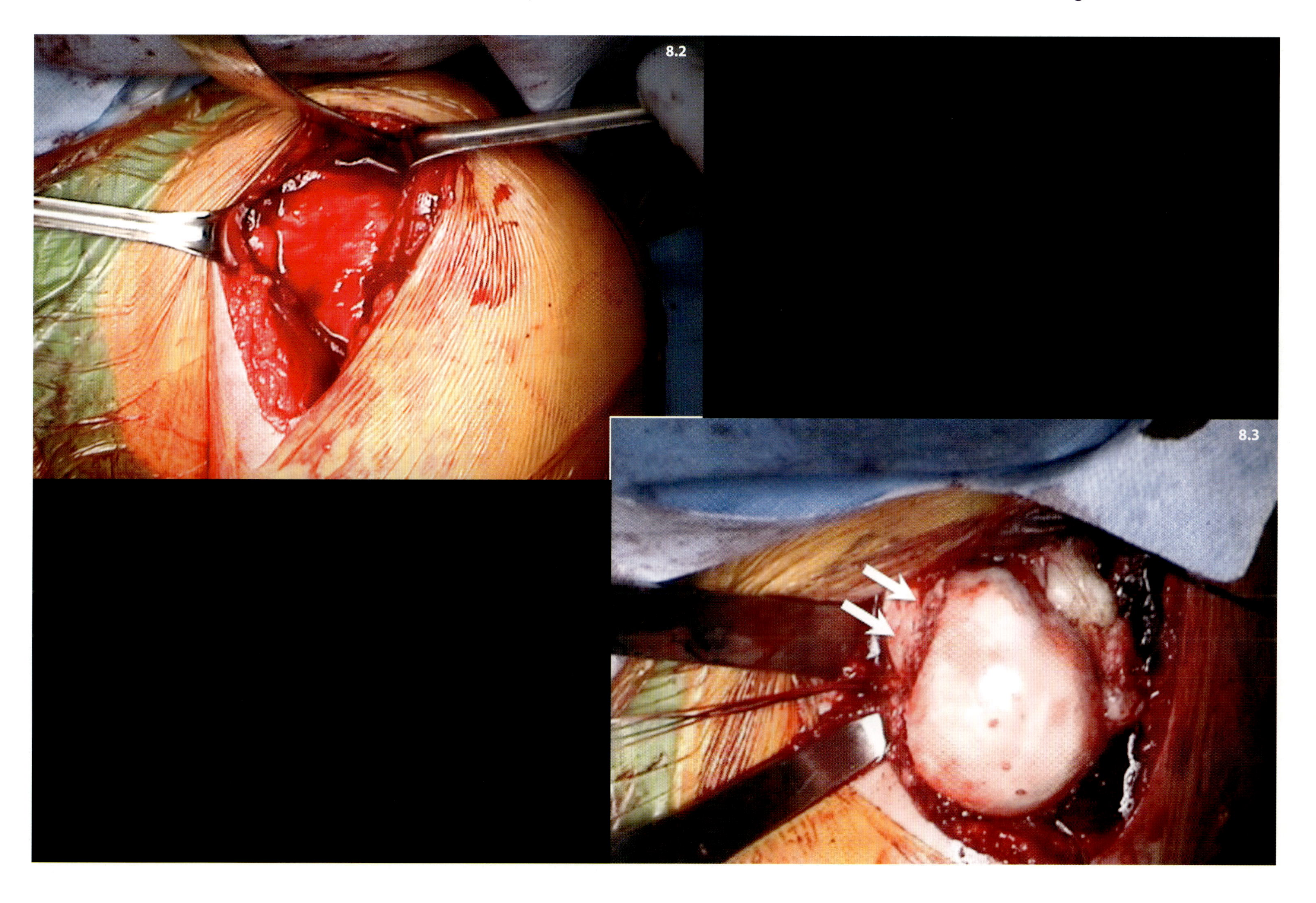
8.2
8.3

drill guide is chosen to ensure defect coverage (Fig. 8.4), and the guidewire is inserted in the center of the defect (Fig. 8.5). A cannulated drill that is present with the instrumentation system is used, and the hole is subsequently tapped to allow insertion of the taper post

Fig. 8.4. Drill guide is placed to ensure complete defect coverage

Fig. 8.5. Guidewire is inserted into the center of the defect

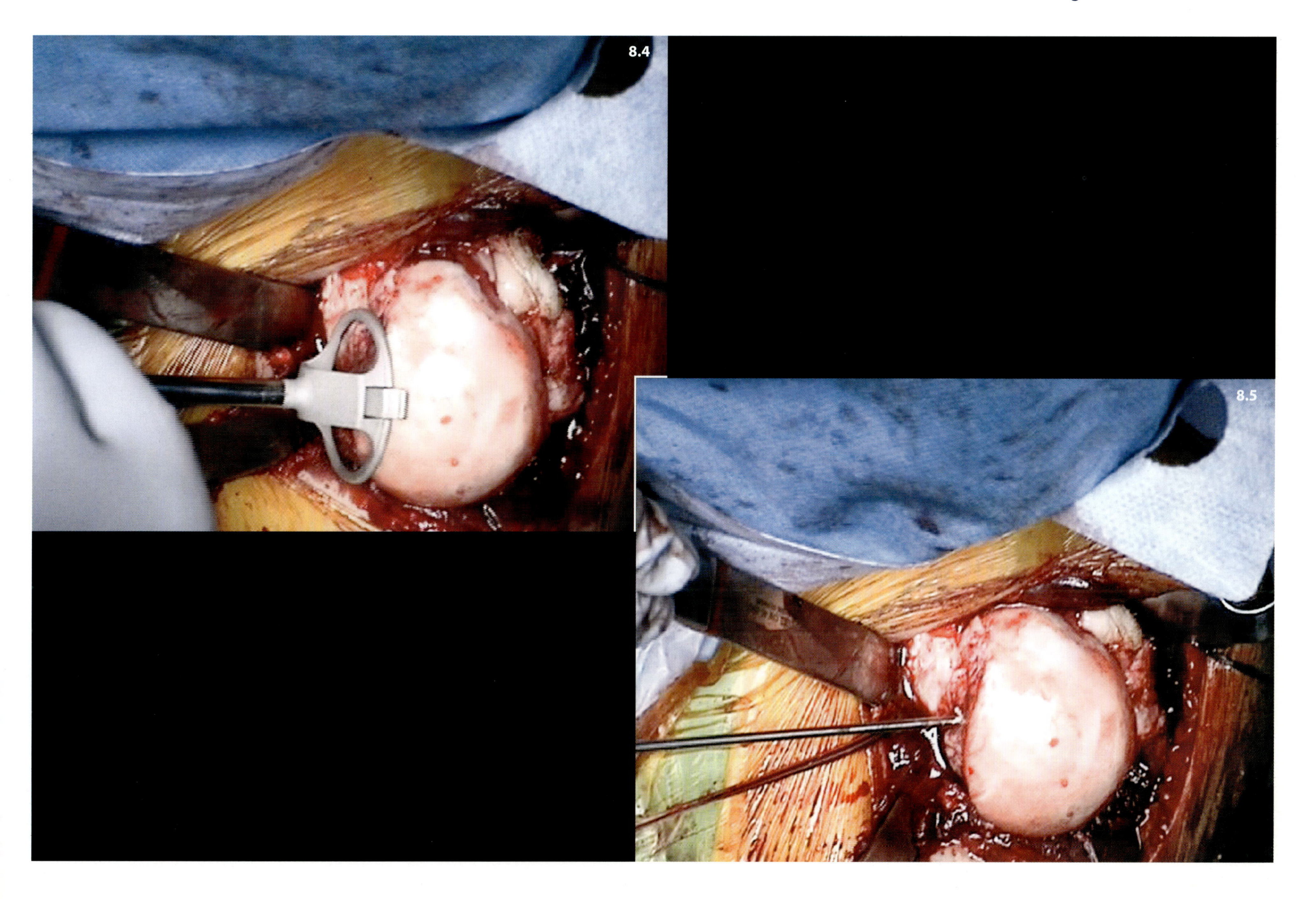
8.4
8.5

(Fig. 8.6). A centering shaft is placed into the taper of the taper post, and a contact probe is used to obtain offsets at the superior/inferior and medial/lateral margins (Fig. 8.7). These are recorded, and using the sizing card that comes with the instrumentation, the appropriate size of the articular component is chosen. The centering shaft and contact probe are removed, and the guide pin is replaced. The circular cutter is inserted over the guide pin to score the articular cartilage to subchondral bone, and the surface reamer (chosen based on

Fig. 8.6. Taper post is inserted

Fig. 8.7. Offset points are obtained using the contact probe

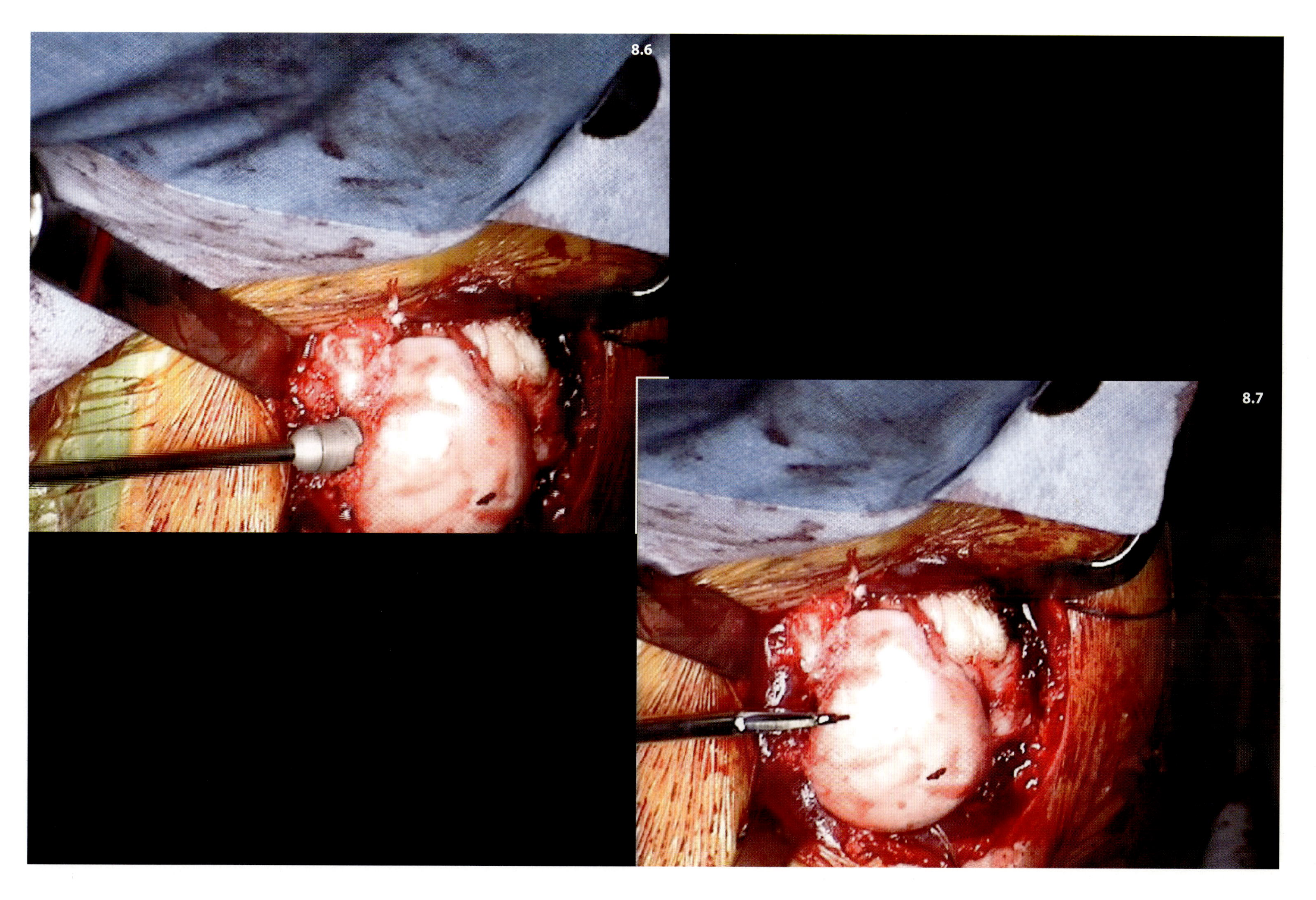
8.6
8.7

previously measured offsets) is used to ream to the taper post (Fig. 8.8). The sizing trial that also matches the previously determined offsets is inserted to ensure the implant is flush with the adjacent articular surface (Fig. 8.9). If it is not congruent, an upsized reamer is used for additional reaming, and the matched sizing trial is used to confirm congruency. The final implant is appropriately positioned

Fig. 8.8. Surface reamer is used to ream to subchondral bone

Fig. 8.9. Trial size is placed

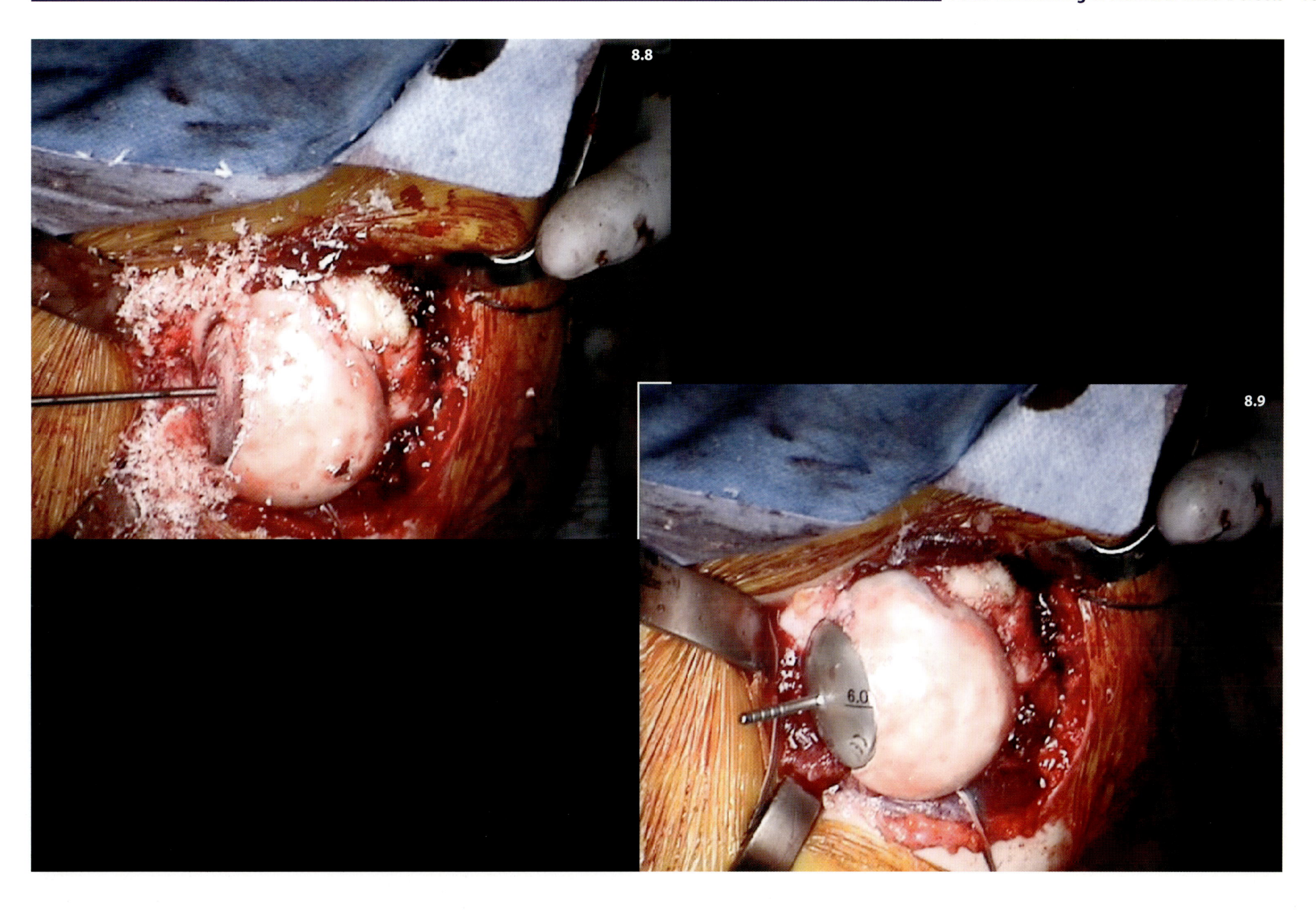
8.8
8.9
6.0

and impacted into place (Fig. 8.10). It should be confirmed again that the component is congruent with the articular surface. The joint is copiously irrigated, and the sutures are tied to complete the labral repair. The capsule is closed in pants-over-vest fashion to reduce any capsular redundancy (Fig. 8.11). The subscapularis is repaired, and the wound is closed in layered fashion.

8.4 Technique: Humeral-head Allograft

As described [19], an extended deltopectoral approach is used similar to the technique described in the previous section. After adequate exposure of the Hill-Sachs lesion, a saw is used to create a chevron-shaped defect that is smoothed with a rasp

Fig. 8.10. Final implant positioned

Fig. 8.11. Capsule is closed

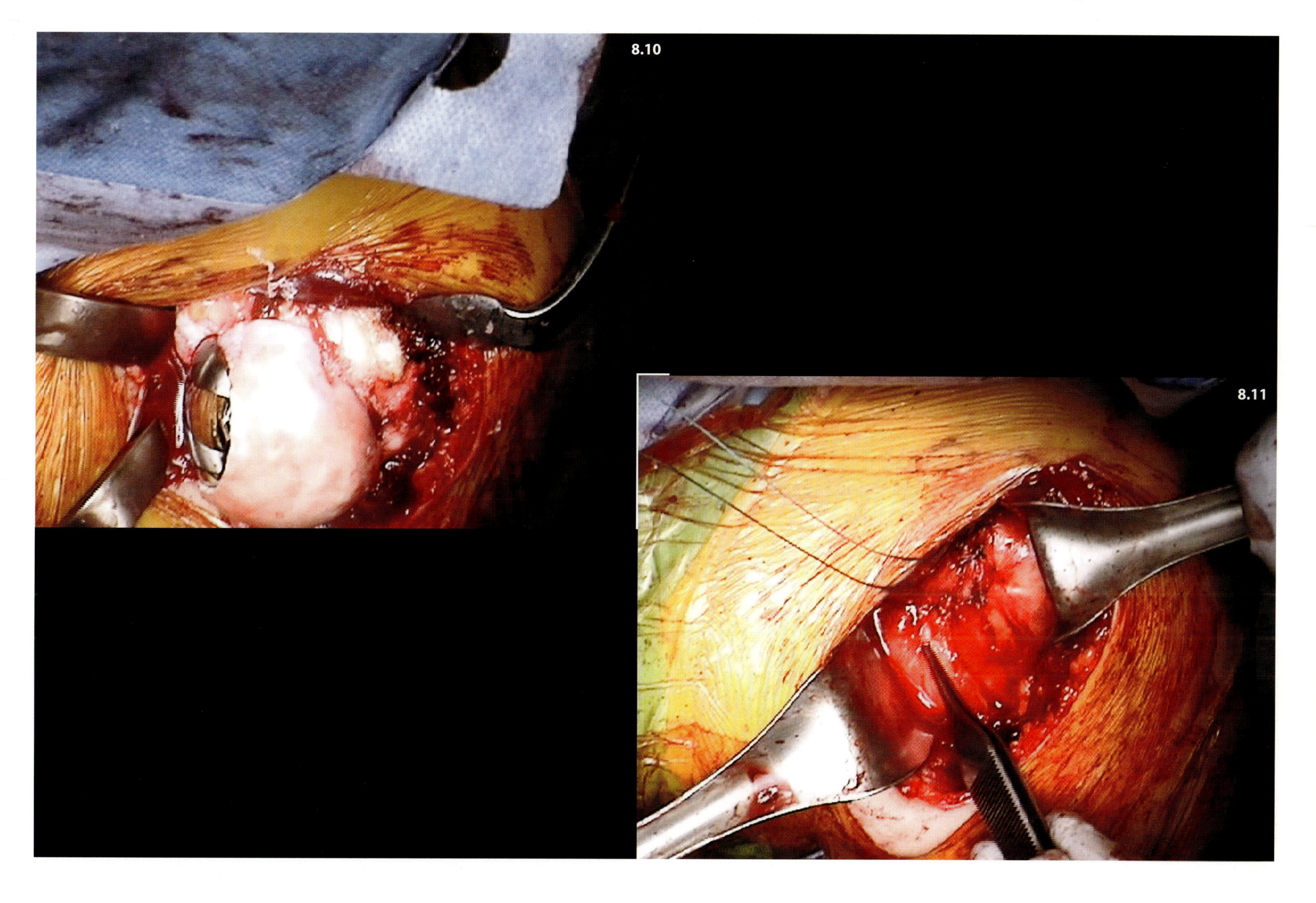
8.10
8.11

(Fig. 8.12). Defect base, height, and length are measured. At this point, a fresh-frozen side- and size-matched humeral-head allograft is used. This typically needs to be requested from a reputable tissue bank. If a matched graft is not available, we use non-matched grafts or femoral heads. Using a matched humeral-head allograft, a chevron-shaped wedge of approximately 2–3 cm larger for each dimension is taken from approximately the same quadrant. This wedge is then placed in the defect and any excess is trimmed so that the graft is press-fit and congruent to the surrounding articular surface. It is provisionally secured in place with 2 or 3 0.045-in. Kirschner wires that are sequentially replaced by 3.5-mm fully threaded cortical screws (Fig. 8.13). The

Fig. 8.12. Hill-Sachs lesion is exposed and prepared for allograft reconstruction

Fig. 8.13. Size-matched humeral-head allograft is positioned and provisionally stabilized with Kirschner wires

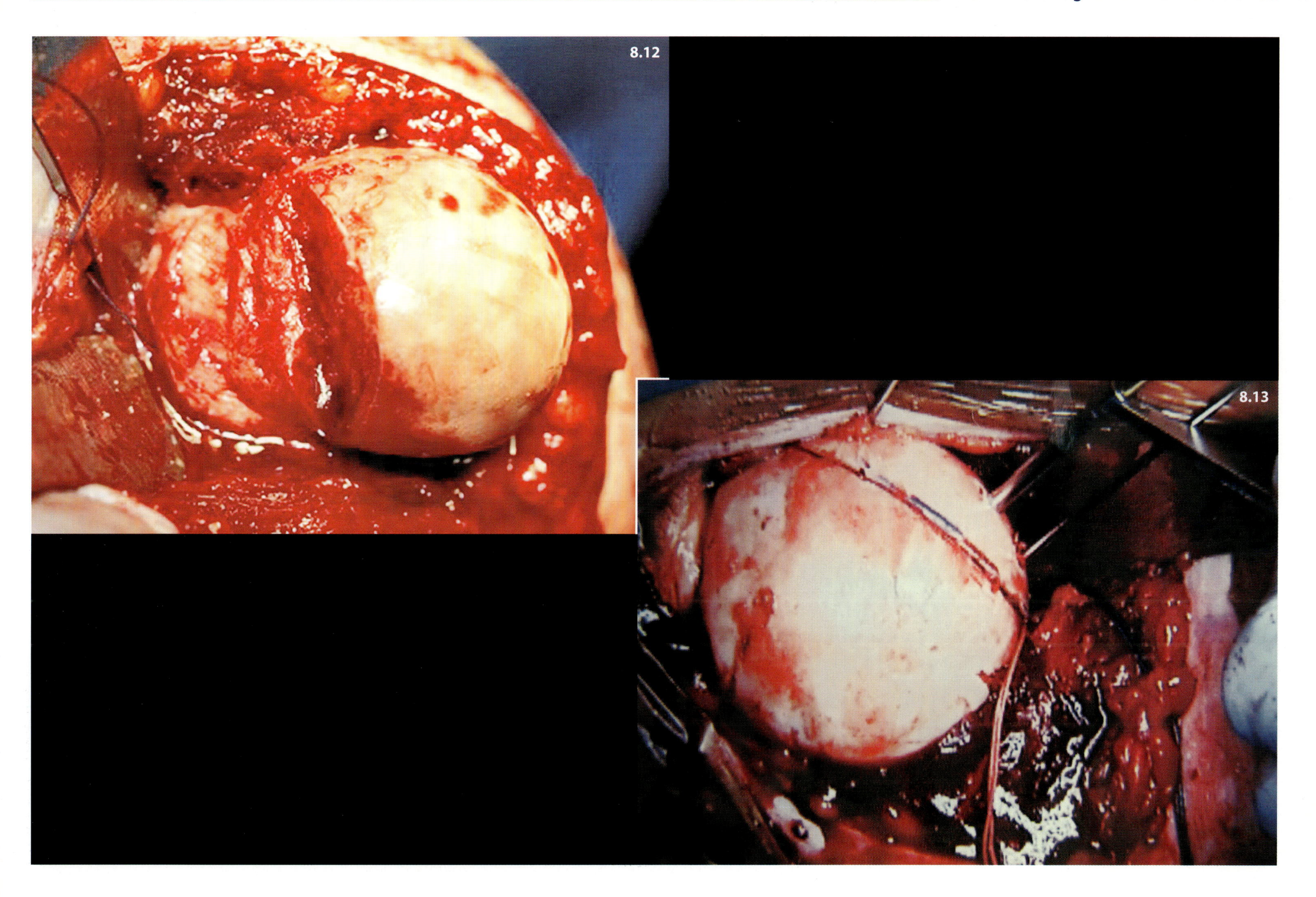
8.12
8.13

screw heads are countersunk below the level of the articular surface (Fig. 8.14). The joint is copiously irrigated, and the wound is closed in a similar fashion as described above.

8.5 Postoperative Rehabilitation

The patient is placed in a sling immediately and pendulum exercises initiated on postoperative day 1. Assisted range of motion to work on forward elevation and external rotation, limited to 20°, is the focus of the initial 6 weeks of rehabilitation. Care is taken to avoid excessive passive external rotation to protect the capsular and subscapularis repair. Assisted internal rotation exercises can be started 2 weeks after surgery. At 6 weeks, patients work on terminal stretching and begin a strengthening program. This is under the guidance of a physical therapist under whose guidance the patient will progress as tolerated. Full range of motion and strength is typically achieved by 6 months.

8.6 Complications

Risk of nerve injury, cephalic-vein injury, and subscapularis rupture inherent risks to the deltopectoral approach exist. No complications have been noted by us after using the HemiCAP implant. Graft resorption, hardware complications, and development of early osteoarthritis has been reported following humeral-head allograft transplantation [19].

8.7 Clinical Results

Literature on the application of resurfacing arthroplasty for humeral-head defects in the face of shoulder instability is scant. This is largely due to the fact that there are no clear criteria for determining clinically significant humeral-head defects. Furthermore, most patients are young, and there is a natural reluctance to place any artificial implant in young patients. Two reports of three cases noted good early results in using the HemiCAP implant for this purpose [9, 20]. To date, we have performed approximately 20 HemiCAP implants, with no recurrent instability (unpublished data). This technique is a promising option for large humeral-head defects associated with shoulder instability, though long-term results remain to be determined.

References

1. Bankart AS, Cantab MC (1993) Recurrent or habitual dislocation of the shoulder-joint. 1923. Clin Orthop Relat Res 291:3-6
2. Bankart ASB (1923) Recurrent or habitual dislocation of the shoulder joint. Br Med J 1:1132
3. Bankart ASB (1938) The pathology and treatment of recurrent dislocation of the shoulder joint. Br J Surg 26:23
4. Lynch JR, Clinton JM, Dewing CB et al (2009) Treatment of osseous defects associated with anterior shoulder instability. J Shoulder Elbow Surg 18:317-328
5. Lenters TR, Franta AK, Wolf FM et al (2007) Arthroscopic compared with open repairs for recurrent anterior shoulder instability. A systematic review and meta-analysis of the literature. J Bone Joint Surg Am 89:244-254
6. Pelet S, Jolles BM, Farron A (2006) Bankart repair for recurrent anterior glenohumeral instability: results at twenty-nine years' follow-up. J Shoulder Elbow Surg 15:203-207
7. Burkhart SS, Danaceau SM (2000) Articular arc length mismatch as a cause of failed bankart repair. Arthroscopy 16:740-744
8. Purchase RJ, Wolf EM, Hobgood ER et al (2008) Hill-Sachs "remplissage": an arthroscopic solution for the engaging Hill-Sachs lesion. Arthroscopy 24:723-726
9. Moros C, Ahmad CS (2009) Partial humeral head resurfacing and Latarjet coracoid transfer for treatment of recurrent anterior glenohumeral instability. Orthopedics 32(8)
10. Chapovsky F, Kelly JD (2005) Osteochondral allograft transplantation for treatment of glenohumeral instability. Arthroscopy 21:1007

Fig. 8.14. Screws are countersunk to avoid hardware irritation on the glenoid

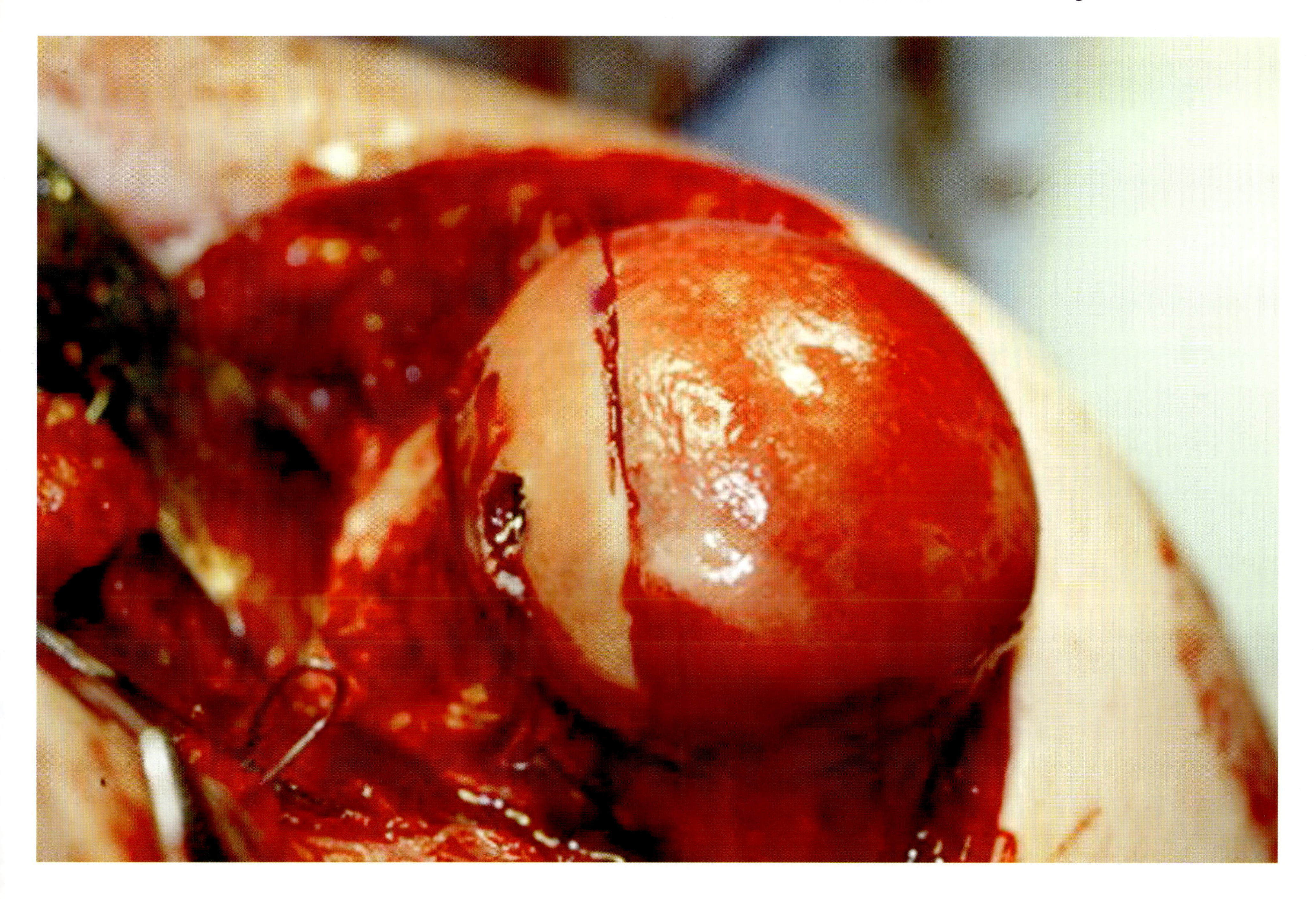

11. Yagishita K, Thomas BJ (2002) Use of allograft for large Hill-Sachs lesion associated with anterior glenohumeral dislocation. A case report. Injury 33:791-794
12. Kropf EJ, Sekiya JK (2007) Osteoarticular allograft transplantation for large humeral head defects in glenohumeral instability. Arthroscopy 23:322 e321-e325
13. Miniaci A, Berlet G, Hand C, Lin A (2008) Segmental humeral head allografts for recurrent anterior instability of the shoulder with large Hill-Sachs defects: a two to 8 year follow up. J Bone Joint Surg Br 90(Supp 1):86
14. Bernageau J, Patte D, Debeyre J, Ferrane J (1976) [Value of the glenoid profil in recurrent luxations of the shoulder]. Rev Chir Orthop Reparatrice Appar Mot 62(2 suppl):142-147
15. Ito H, Shirai Y, Takayama A, Shibasaki T (1996) A new radiographic projection for the posterolateral notch in cases of recurrent dislocation of the shoulder. Nippon Ika Daigaku Zasshi 63:499-501
16. Kralinger FS, Golser K, Wischatta R et al (2002) Predicting recurrence after primary anterior shoulder dislocation. Am J Sports Med 30:116-120
17. Sekiya JK, Wickwire AC, Stehle JH, Debski RE (2009) Hill-Sachs defects and repair using osteoarticular allograft transplantation: biomechanical analysis using a joint compression model. Am J Sports Med 37:2459-2466
18. Kaar SG, Fening SD, Jones MH et al (2010) Effect of humeral head defect size on glenohumeral stability: a cadaveric study of simulated Hill-Sachs defects. Am J Sports Med 38:594-599
19. Miniaci A, Gish MW (2004) Management of anterior glenohumeral instability associated with large Hill-Sachs defects. Techniques in shoulder & elbow surgery 5:170-175
20. Grodin P, Leith J (2009) Combined large Hill-Sachs and bony Bankart lesions treated by Latarjet and partial humeral head resurfacing: a report of 2 cases. Can J Surg 52:249-254

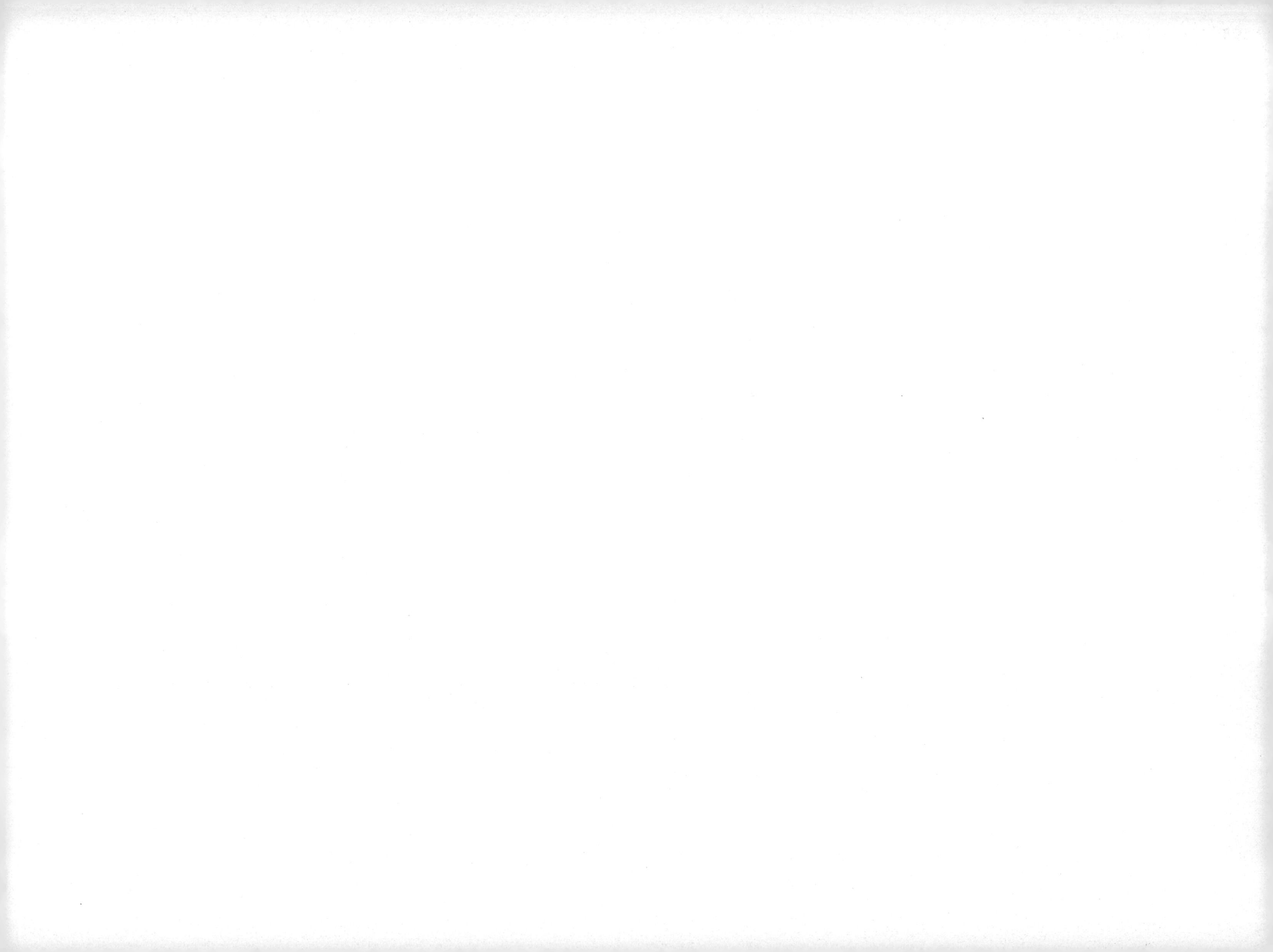

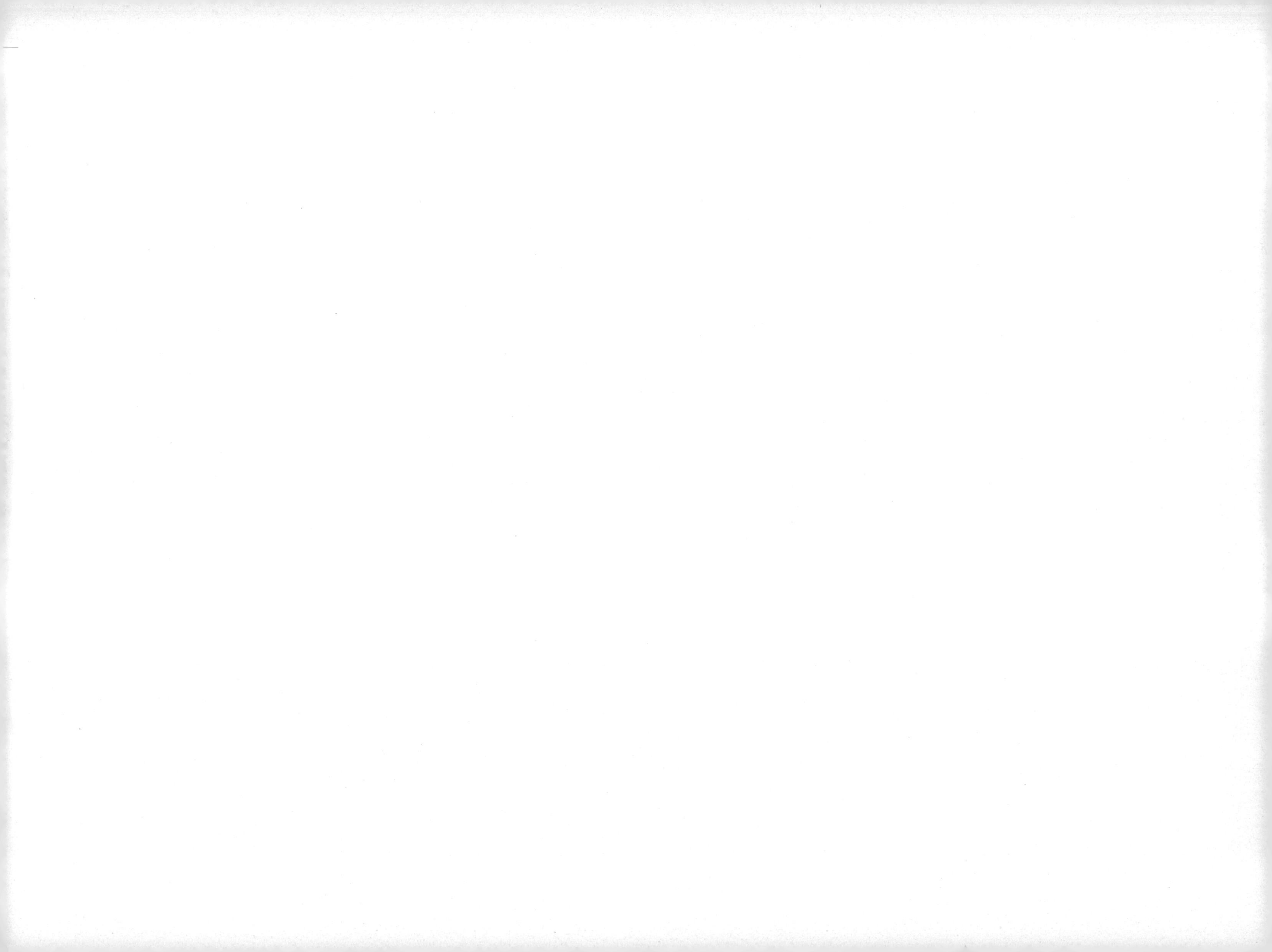

Printed in May 2011